ELLIE HERMAN'S

PILATES
REFORMER

SECOND EDITION

ELLIE HERMAN BOOKS, BROOKLYN

Published in the United States by
Ellie Herman Books
788A Union Street
Brooklyn, NY 11215
www.elliehermanpilates.com

ISBN 978-0-9765181-0-5

Ellie Herman, co-author
Susi May, co-author
Lisa Graham, contributing author, copy editor, 2nd edition
Jenny Belluomini, copy editor
Elizabeth Gand, copy editor

Design & composition by Margaret Banda & SeMe Sung

Printed in Canada by
Transcontinental Printing

Please Note:
This book has been written and published strictly for informational purposes, and in no way should be used as a substitute for consultation with health care professionals. You should not consider educational material herein to be the practice of medicine or to replace consultation with a physician or other medical practitioner. The author and publisher are providing you with information in this work so that you can have the knowledge and can choose, at your own risk, to act on that knowledge. The author and publisher also urge all readers to be aware of their health status and to consult health care professionals before beginning any health program.

ALSO BY ELLIE HERMAN

Pilates Mat

Pilates Springboard

Pilates Cadillac

Pilates Wunda Chair

Pilates Props Workbook

Pilates Workbook on the Ball

Pilates for Dummies

CONTENTS

CONTENTS CONTINUED

THE REFORMER

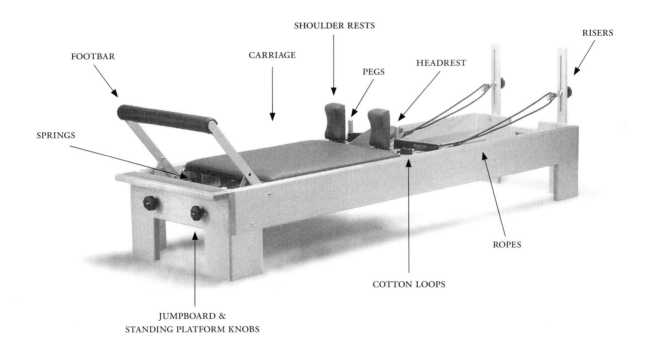

SHOULDER RESTS

RISERS

FOOTBAR

CARRIAGE

PEGS

HEADREST

SPRINGS

ROPES

COTTON LOOPS

JUMPBOARD &
STANDING PLATFORM KNOBS

THE REFORMER

The Reformer is probably the most popular piece of Pilates equipment. It has the most repertoire, is the most versatile, and it's just plain fun. Below are some important things to understand when using the Reformer...

HOME: Home refers to the position when the carriage is in its Starting Position; i.e. the carriage is "home."

SPRING SETTINGS: The spring settings in this book are based on a person between 125–150 pounds. If you are significantly smaller or larger than this, you need to adjust your springs accordingly. For control exercises, lessening the weight will increase the challenge. Using second gear is another way to decrease resistance.

RISERS: Standard position for risers is down, but you can raise the ropes any time you want to decrease the load challenge (i.e. Kneeling Side Arm Series), or if you do a Rowing exercise up on the long box instead of seated on the carriage. Also, rising the risers up for the Leg Series allows for greater Range of Motion of the legs without hitting the ropes.

STANDARD LENGTH ROPES: For most exercises, measure the ropes to fit tightly around the shoulder rests. Once you've measured them, you can remove them and leave them around the "pegs" so that they are out of your way.

LONG ROPES: For *Long Spine* and Leg Series, lengthen the ropes so that the "D" ring is centered between the shoulder rests. This lengthens the ropes about 6–8" longer than standard length.

SHORT ROPES: For *Roll Downs*, shorten the ropes so that the end of the foot loops are at the head rest. For *Hamstrings* go a little shorter.

BALANCED BODY FOOTBARS: The *Studio Reformer* pictured has a standard footbar with 3 settings; high bar, low bar, and bar down. Balanced Body also manufactures specialty footbars which offer flexibility for clients of different heights. Their Revo Footbar locks into place to allow clients to pull on the bar while on the machine. The Revo also allows lets you move the "home" away with the spring bar, which allows taller people to start exercises with the same resistance as everyone else.

The Infinity Footbar includes the Revo spring bar system, making it the most versatile footbar on the market. The Infinity Footbar adjusts along the whole length of the Reformer, allowing clients of all heights to gain the same benefits from the exercises. This is really great for tall people, short people and children. The Infinity Footbar also offers more high/low adjustability which allows for some fun variations on some of the exercises (i.e. Stomach Massage Series can be done with the footbar slightly lower than the standard low bar).

AN INTRODUCTION TO ELLIE HERMAN

I discovered Pilates many moons ago when I was a professional dancer and choreographer in San Francisco circa 1988. But my work with *The Flying Buttresses* performance troupe did not garner enough cash to support my bohemian lifestyle in the Bay Area. And being twenty-two, full of hubris, and an experience junkie to boot, I did what every self-respecting young woman in my position would do: I became a professional wrestler. My career as "Ruth Less" was cut short during a tag team match when a tough cookie tried to take me down. I stood my ground just long enough to hear a loud "snapping" sound: my anterior cruciate ligament, torn, completely. I figured my dance career was over for sure. And by losing the fight, I'd just missed out on what should've been an easy 200 bucks.

Enter Pilates. At St. Francis Hospital in San Francisco, I began treatment in a Dance Medicine department dedicated to Pilates-based rehabilitation. After six months under the care of Elizabeth Larkham, I returned to dancing. I then realized that Pilates had not only allowed me to resume jumping, leaping, and twirling—it had actually improved my technique, control, balance, and core strength.

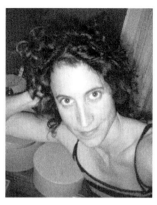

ELLIE HERMAN

I then moved to New York City, where I enrolled in the MFA dance program at New York University. I took morning Pilates mat classes with Kathy Grant, one of Joseph Pilates' original disciples. Kathy taught me how depth and creativity could be brought to the Pilates Method, while helping to relieve the mounting hip pain I was experiencing due to daily ballet classes. I decided to stop pirouetting my way to early arthritis, and instead began a Pilates teacher training program with Romana Kyranowska, another of Joe Pilates' original students.

I returned to San Francisco in 1992 and the following year opened a studio in the Mission district of San Francisco. In 2001, I began a second studio in Oakland, California. I sold those studios, returned to New York, and have owned and operated Ellie Herman Studio in Park Slope, Brooklyn since 2005.

I developed a system called *Walk-ilates,* which uses MBT shoes to blend core strength with gait and posture. I designed a piece of Pilates equipment called the Pilates Springboard, an inexpensive and space-saving variation of the Wall Unit/Cadillac.

I've authored eight books to date including professional manuals for Pilates Mat, Physioball, Props and every major piece of Pilates equipment, and I wrote "Pilates for Dummies." I also have a Master of Science degree in Acupuncture and Chinese Herbal Medicine from the American College of Traditional Chinese Medicine in San Francisco.

Please check **www.elliehermanpilates.com** for the latest news on my studio and other adventures in Pilates. I am available for workshops and teacher trainings. Contact me at **ellie@elliehermanpilates.com**.

THE SKINNY ON MR. PILATES

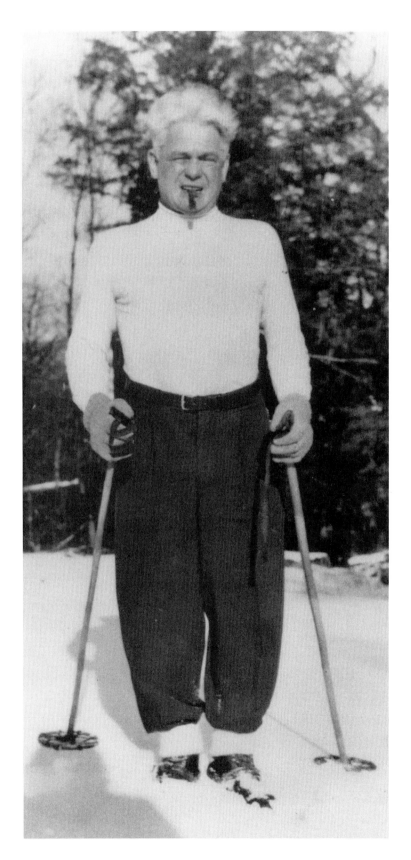

Joseph Hubertus Pilates was born in Germany in 1880, and as a young man suffered from asthma and poor health. Over his lifetime, he overcame his frailties and became an accomplished athlete—an avid skier, diver, gymnast, yogi, and pugilist.

Mr. Pilates was a visionary who had overarching ideas about how to be a healthy happy human. He first developed a series of exercises to be done on a mat designed to build abdominal strength and overall body control. He then invented various pieces of equipment to enhance the results of his expanding repertoire of exercises. The apocryphal story goes that Joseph Pilates was a nurse stationed in an English internment camp during WWI, and he had the bright idea to rig springs above hospital beds, which allowed patients to rehabilitate their injuries and to exercise while lying on their backs. This bed-like set-up later evolved into the Cadillac, one of the main pieces of Pilates equipment.

In 1923 Joseph Pilates emigrated to the United States, settling in New York City, where he opened a studio on Eighth Avenue in Manhattan and started training and rehabilitating professional dancers including George Balanchine and Martha Graham.

In his book *Return to Life,* Joseph Pilates lays out a whole regime to improve overall health, including of course, the classical Pilates Mat exercises, with Joe himself pictured going through the whole series (worth seeing!). He originally called his method "Contrology" and only after he taught his method to others was it referred to as "Pilates." In his book he states, [Contrology] "develops the body uniformly, corrects wrong postures, restores physical vitality, invigorates the mind, and elevates the spirit."

Over his lifetime, Pilates invented over 20 contraptions some of which look a little like medieval torture devices—constructed of wood and metal piping, using a variable combination of pulleys, straps, bars, boxes, and springs. The total Pilates repertoire consists of over 500 exercises, including Pilates Mat, Reformer, Cadillac, Wunda Chair, Spine Corrector, Ladder Barrel, and Tower.

THE PILATES LINEAGE

The original Eighth Avenue Pilates studio in Manhattan bore the first generation of Pilates teachers: Romana Kyranowska, Kathy Grant, Ron Fletcher, Eve Gentry, Carola Trier, Mary Bowen, and Bruce King. Some of these protégés branched out and opened studios around the country, while others stayed in New York City. Romana remained in Joe's original studio until after his death. Kathy Grant still practices in a small studio above the NYU dance department, where I was fortunate enough to have been graced by her presence. For the last 50 years, the Pilates Method has been passed down through many more generations of teachers and the Method has transformed a great deal along the way. Many modern Pilates teachers now bring their own insights to improve the original, while others cling to the notion of a "pure" Pilates which, in their mind should not be trifled with! In my opinion, if Mr. Pilates was an innovator, and within his own lifetime changed and evolved his repertoire and invented new contraptions, why shouldn't we?

WHAT EXACTLY IS PILATES?

Pilates exercises as a whole develop strong abdominal, back, butt, and deep postural muscles to support the skeletal system and act as what Pilates called the "powerhouse" of the body. The Pilates Method works to strengthen the center, lengthen the spine, increase body awareness, build muscle tone, and gain flexibility. The Pilates Method is also an excellent rehabilitation system for back, knee, hip, shoulder, and repetitive stress injuries. Pilates addresses the body as a whole, correcting the body's asymmetries and chronic weaknesses to prevent re-injury and bring the body back into balance.

EIGHT PRINCIPLES OF PILATES

Joseph Pilates' book, *Return to Life,* maps out the eight important principles that underlie the Pilates Method. These concepts are the backbone of the Pilates Method.

CONTROL

A fundamental rule when doing Pilates: Control your body's every movement! This rule applies not only to the exercises themselves but also to transitions between exercises, how you get on and off the equipment, and your overall attention to detail while working out. When doing mat exercises, Control comes into play with the attack and ending of each movement. When the body puts on the brakes in a controlled manner, it is training the muscles to work as they lengthen. This is called eccentric muscle contraction, which builds long and flexible muscles. Also, when focusing on Control of a movement, the body is forced to recruit helper muscles (we call these synergists), which are usually smaller than the main muscles. When many muscles work together to do one movement, or when muscles work synergistically, the body as a whole develops greater balance and coordination. Also, the big muscles won't bulk up because they don't have to do all the work by themselves. Thus we become a long and lean machine. Once your body learns to move with Control you will feel more confident doing all kinds of things from skiing that advanced run, to tango dancing, or to climbing a ladder to get up to that rocking roof deck party.

BREATH

Most people do not utilize their full lung capacity. Shallow Breathing is an unfortunate side effect of a sedentary and stressful life. Also, as a Pilates instructor it's painful to see how people often hold their breath when performing a new or difficult task. I often have to tell my clients to exhale, because otherwise they won't! Some people will actually get out of breath during a new exercise merely because they haven't exhaled. When you hold your breath, you tense muscles that can ultimately exacerbate improper posture and reinforce tension habits. That is why consistent Breathing is essential to flowing movement and proper muscle balance. As with yoga, Breathing is an essential part of the Pilates Method and distinguishes it from other exercise forms.

Every Pilates exercise has a specific Breathing pattern assigned to it. Breathing while moving is not always an easy assignment, but when accomplished, beautiful things can happen. Focused Breath can help maximize the body's ability to stretch, and through this release of tension you will gain optimal body Control. Deep inhalation and full exhalation also exercises the lungs and increases lung capacity, bringing deep relaxation as a pleasant side effect.

FLOWING MOVEMENT

If you look at photographs of Pilates exercises, you might notice the similarity to many yoga postures. But unlike yoga, we do not hold positions in Pilates—instead we Flow from one movement to another. When doing a Pilates workout, you want to Flow and move freely during the movement phase and finish with control and precision. Flowing Movement integrates the nervous system, the muscles, and the joints, and trains the body to move smoothly and evenly.

PRECISION

Precision is similar to Control with the added element of spatial awareness. When attacking any movement you must know exactly where that movement starts and ends. All Pilates exercises have precise definitions of where the body should be at all times: the angle of the legs, the placement of the elbows, the positioning of the head and neck, even what the fingers are doing! The little things count in Pilates.

CENTERING

Sometimes after a long day of training clients, I can hear a tape running inside my head that says, "pull the navel to the spine...." Why? Because I have repeated this mantra all day to cue my clients to scoop in their bellies. All exercises should be done with the deep abdominals engaged to ensure proper Centering. Most Pilates exercises focus on developing abdominal strength either directly or indirectly. Even when performing an exercise that focuses on strengthening the arm muscles, you should keep your Abdominal Scoop, keep your shoulders pulling down the back, and perhaps even squeeze your butt. All these actions promote Centering and core muscle strength. No exercise should be done to the detriment of core stabilization. In other words, if your spine moves like a noodle when it should be a rock-hard *Plank*, then you are not allowed to progress to the next level of an exercise.

STABILITY

Pilates exercises utilize the concept of Stability—whether it be torso Stability, shoulder Stability or ankle Stability—which is the key to health for your spine and joints. After an injury, there will generally be instability in the affected area. The first thing you want to do is learn to stabilize the injured part so as to prevent re-injury and to allow the healing process to begin. Thus Pilates is one of the safest forms of exercise to do after injury. Pilates will also prevent injury, for if you have Stability in your torso and joints, you are much less likely to injure yourself in the first place.

RANGE OF MOTION

"Range of Motion" is a phrase used by medical professionals to describe the movement of a joint. For instance, the Range of Motion of your shoulder joint is defined by how high you can raise your arm in front of you, behind you, etc. Range of Motion can be affected by the length or tightness in your muscles and other tissues such as ligaments and fascia (connective tissue). Basically, Range of Motion is just another way of describing flexibility. If you lack flexibility in your joints or spine, then Pilates can increase Range of Motion. But if you have too much Range of Motion, which causes instability in the joints and spine, then Pilates exercises will teach you how to stabilize those areas. This is how Pilates brings balance to the body. It is important to understand how to limit your Range of Motion if you lack Stability because this will help to prevent injury in the future.

OPPOSITION

Down to go up. Up to go down. When teaching Pilates I often use imagery that uses the concept of Opposition to enhance the form of the exercise. For instance, when doing a *Roll Down*, which starts seated and upright, I'll always say, "imagine you have a golden string lifting you up from the back of the top of your head as you roll down your spine...." This gives the client the idea to lift up really tall before flexing and rolling back. Basically, going up as they go down. This lengthens the spine and takes the compression out of flexing the spine. This is essential to keeping the spine healthy and injury free. Opposition can be used in many ways to get better form from your clients.

ELLIE'S NINTH PRINCIPLE: BODY AWARENESS

Most of us never learned how to live in our bodies. We don't really know how to sit, stand or walk properly, and we certainly don't know how to fix ourselves once we are broken. Pilates can teach you all this. That's why I call it "high exercise"—because it teaches us the fundamentals of how to take care of our spine, joints, and muscles. It teaches us how to not hurt ourselves and how to get the most longevity from our physical beings.

Many clients have told me that they can hear my voice in their head saying things like, "...relax your shoulders, lengthen through the back of your neck, scoop your belly in."

If you suffer from pain because of faulty postural habits that you aren't even aware of, after a few good sessions with a competent Pilates instructor you will be pleasantly surprised by how fast a newfound awareness can affect a positive change in your body.

ELLIE HERMAN'S PILATES ALPHABET

Just as every word can be broken down into letters, so can every Pilates exercise be broken down into discrete parts. The Pilates alphabet is my way to facilitate the learning process and de-mystify even the most complex Pilates exercises. Almost every advanced exercise contains basic movements that repeat over and over in the repertoire.

ABDOMINAL SCOOP

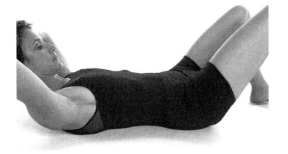

"Pull the navel in toward the spine...." I've probably said that phrase over a million times in my life. It is the first, middle and last cue in the Pilates Method. The Abdominal Scoop can be done anywhere and at any time, and frankly it should be done as much as possible. Anatomically, "the scoop" engages your deepest abdominal muscles, which function to hold in your viscera and, when contracted, decrease the diameter of the abdominal wall. The Abdominal Scoop works a lot like a drawstring around a pair of sweat pants when pulled taut. You have four layers of abdominal muscles; your deepest one is called the transversus abdominis. The second and third layers are called your internal and external obliques. And the most superficial abdominal layer is called your rectus abdominis. The rectus (as we call it in the biz) is a workaholic muscle and will do all the work if you let it. The Abdominal Scoop, or "navel to spine" image is meant to bring in the deeper three layers, which work to compress the abdominal wall and help support

the back. In every exercise you want to be using your Abdominal Scoop to get the most profound results possible. Pooching is the opposite of scooping, so no pooching allowed!

BALANCE POINT

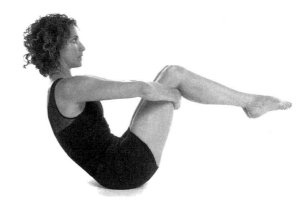

Balance Point, in my vocabulary, is both a position and a fundamental mat exercise. As a position, it where you begin and end the rolling exercises in the Mat, and it is also the place you arrive at the top of the *Teaser*. You can practice *Balance Point* by sitting up with your knees bent, holding on to the backs of your thighs. Roll back slightly behind your tailbone, pull your belly in, and lift your feet off the floor. In order to maintain your balance and stop yourself from roll-ing backward, you must engage and pull in your deep abdominal muscles and slightly round the low back. This teaches you that to balance with ease, you must engage your deep abdominals.

BRIDGE

Bridge is a both a basic position in Pilates that we come in and out of, as well as a beginning level exer-cise on the mat and the ball. In kinesiological terms, a *Bridge* is extension of the hips. In lay terms, this means lifting your hips up off the floor, using your butt and hamstrings. I want to point out that a *Bridge* should be done from the hip extensors (butt and hamstrings) and not from the back muscles. Therefore when doing a *Bridge* you must keep your spine neutral (or even slightly flexed) but and make sure to definite-ly not extend (arch) the spine! This is not Yoga!

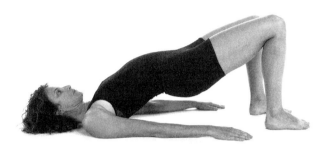

CORRECT BRIDGE: THE BACK IS NEUTRAL

INCORRECT BRIDGE: THE BACK IS HYPEREXTENDED

C-CURVE

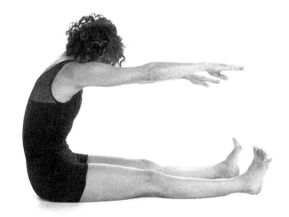

Martha Graham, the mother of Modern Dance, introduced spinal flexion, (or what she termed "the contraction") which revolutionized dance. It was a primal, dark, and oh-so-human movement. Joe Pilates worked with Graham in his Eighth Avenue studio and, I suspect, learned a couple of tricks from her. (Who knows—maybe she learned them from him?) The C-Curve is rounding of the back, or flexion of the spine. The "C" is meant to describe the shape of the back after you scoop in your belly. This shape should always be initiated by your deep Abdominal Scoop and should provide a lovely stretch for your spine. Many Pilates exercises use the C-Curve.

DOOR FRAME ARMS

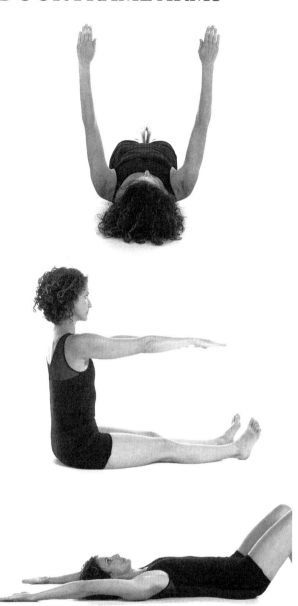

DOOR FRAME ARMS: 3 WAYS

Arms are straight, shoulder distance apart, making the shape of the outer frame of a door. This describes the shape of your arms in many Pilates exercises, whether your arms are above your head, by your sides when lying supine on the floor, or supporting you in a *Plank* position.

HIP UP

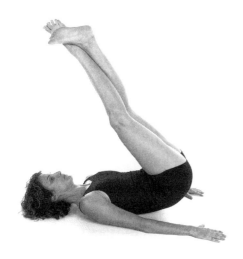

The name says it all. Lie on your back with your legs up, your knees bent, and your Door Frame Arms down by your sides. Rock back and lift your hips up by using your low Abdominal Scoop. The Hip Up works your lower abdominals and can be very challenging for those with a weak low abdominals, a tight back, or a large butt!

LEVITATION

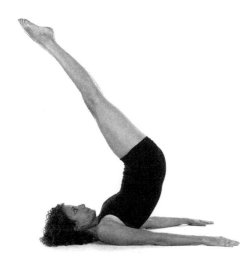

When you combine a Hip Up with hip extension, you get Levitation. Try it if you like: lie on your back, lift up your hips with your Abdominal Scoop, and at the top of the Hip Up, squeeze your butt. You'll feel your hips levitate, rising perceptibly higher, as if the hand of the Pilates Goddess came down and lifted your hips magically and effortlessly off the floor.

PILATES ABDOMINAL POSITIONING

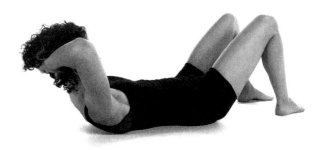

The Pilates Abdominal Positioning is my way to describe the placement of the upper body when performing many of the supine Pilates floor exercises. When lying on your back (supine), lift your head off the floor just high enough so that the bottom tips of your shoulder blades are either just touching or just off the floor. Imagine that the base of the sternum is anchored to the floor and the back of the neck and upper back are stretching around that anchor. Make sure to keep a space the size of a tangerine under your chin (see below); you are not meant to over-stretch the back of your neck. It is essential to maintain this position when performing abdominal exercises. If you allow the head to drop back you will begin to feel fatigue in the neck and you will not be using your abdominals as much. The upper abdominals should be working to maintain this position, and that's where you should feel the burn.

PILATES "V" (PILATES FIRST POSITION)

First Position in dance means standing with your legs together and turned out from the hip, knees facing away from each other, and feet making a "V" shape. The Pilates "V" is very much the same except you never want to force the turn out. Your feet should be making a small "V" shape, like a slice of pie, a nice small Pilates-sized slice. In Pilates we use this First Position in many exercises because external rotation of the hips engages the gluteus maximus and the inner thigh muscles, which helps to stabilize the pelvis and spine. (See Parallel vs. Turn Out in the General Movement Vocabulary section.)

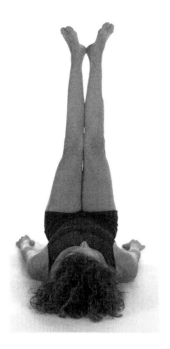

ROSEBUD

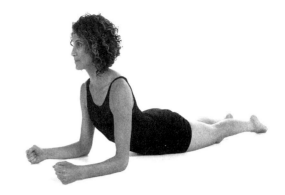

CORRECT NECK PLACEMENT: ROSEBUD ATOP STEM

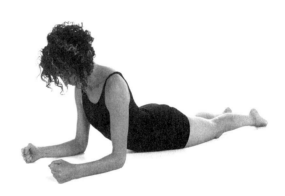

BROKEN BUD: TOO MUCH FLEXION

SERAPE

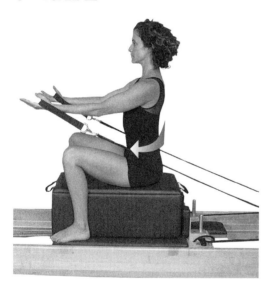

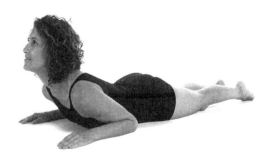

BROKEN BUD: TOO MUCH EXTENSION

A Serape is a shawl that wraps around your body from the back to the front. This is an image we use in my studios to describe the connection of the shoulder blades pulling down the back as you lift your arms forward—as in *Teaser*. The fibers of the serratus anterior and the obliques interdigitate, connecting the back to the front. Think: "down to go up" as you lift your arms, as if they emanate from the upper back.

In every bunch of roses, there always seems to be one with a broken bud—that sad rose that hangs down from the stem. If you imagine your head as the bud and your spine as the stem in a healthy unbroken rose, then in any movement of your spine, your head will follow and continue the curve of the spine without a break. When you move your head in a "faulty" sequence (say, when you come up into a *Swan* or perform back extension from lying on your belly), your head can look like a broken bud; that is, your neck is bent at a greater angle than the rest of your spine. We want no broken buds in Pilates—only healthy long stem roses.

SQUEEZE A TANGERINE

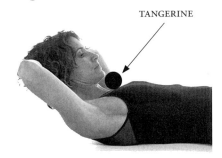

TANGERINE

This is an image that describes the sequencing of your head as you lift it off the floor in flexion. First you should do a small head nod, bring the chin in toward the chest (but don't "juice your tangerine"—keep a small space under your chin) before lifting your head off the floor. The muscle sequencing should be: first your deep neck flexors should fire to nod your head down slightly, then the abdominals lift the head off the mat. The tangerine is the perfect size to image the correct distance your chin should be from your chest when holding your Pilates Abdominal Positioning.

TABLE TOP LEGS

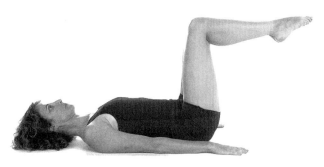

Table Top Legs describes the position of your legs when you are lying supine (on your back), with the knees and feet up off the floor, inner thighs pulling together, knees bent at a 90° angle, and the thighs at a 90° angle to the floor.

STACKING THE SPINE

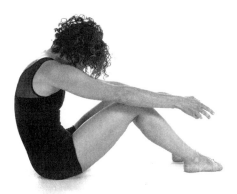

STACKING THE SPINE 1

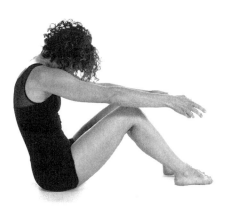

STACKING THE SPINE 2

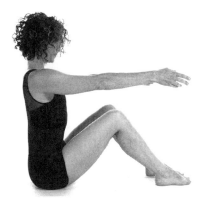

STACKING THE SPINE 3

Stacking the Spine is the ending to a few exercises in the Pilates Method. Stacking the Spine teaches spinal articulation as well as how to sit up vertically. It is a way to sit up or stand erect from a flexed position. Stacking the Spine teaches sequencing from the tail to the head. You start usually from a C-Curve and then stack up from the base of the spine, one vertebra at a time, with the head staying heavy and dropped until the very end. The spine should be completely vertical at the end, with the natural curves of the back in place. (This can be practiced against a wall to better feel the vertical alignment of the spine.)

THORACIC SHELF

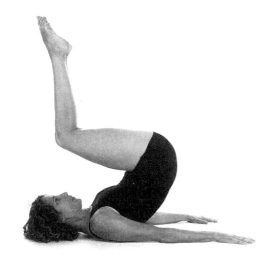

CORRECT NECK PLACEMENT:
BALANCE BETWEEN YOUR SHOULDER BLADES
ON YOUR "THORACIC SHELF"

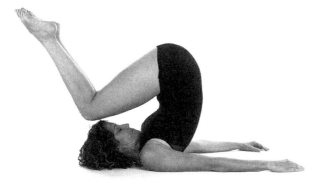

INCORRECT NECK PLACEMENT:
DON'T ROLL ONTO YOUR NECK

This describes the place you want to balance when you are doing all supine inversions that require you to roll onto your upper back. In other words, balance on your shoulder blades, not your neck. This is difficult for people with a tight thoracic spine.

GENERAL MOVEMENT VOCABULARY

ARTICULATION

This is another word for Range of Motion. We use this word mainly when referring to moving the spine one vertebra at a time while rounding down the mat, as opposed to coming down in one piece.

ASIS (ANTERIOR SUPERIOR ILIAC SPINE)

ASIS refers to the bony protrusions at the front the pelvis, palpable in standing and even more visible when supine. They are great bony landmarks to monitor pelvic alignment.

CONTINUOUS BREATHING

Breathe by inhaling and exhaling in an even rhythm rather than coordinating the breath with specific body movements.

EXTENSION

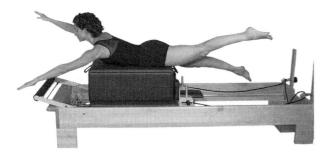

EXTENSION OF THE SPINE, HIPS, KNEES AND ANKLES

Technically, Extension is a movement that brings a part of the body backward from its normal anatomical position, but we also use Extension to mean *to straighten*—as in "straighten your knee." It can also mean *to lengthen* or *stretch*, as in "extend you arms and legs long on the mat." Extension of the spine means the spine is arched back, opening the belly, while the head or tail move backward or toward each other; the *Swan* movement is a perfect example of this principle.

FLEXION

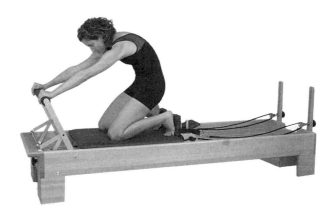

FLEXION OF THE SPINE, HIPS, KNEES AND ANKLES

Flexion is the opposite of Extension: it's a movement that brings a part of the body forward from its normal anatomical position. It also means *to bend*, as in "flex your knee." Flexion of the spine is the movement that brings the head forward (closer) to the pelvis or vice versa; the C-Curve or any abdominal curving is a good example.

PARALLEL VS. TURN OUT

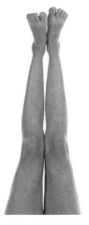

PARALLEL LEGS

If you've ever taken a modern dance class then you probably have heard the terms Parallel legs and Turned Out legs. Simply put, Parallel means your legs are neutral, with knees facing forward as most of

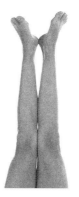

TURNED OUT LEGS; PILATES FIRST POSITION

us do naturally when we stand. Turn Out or external rotation of the hips means your knees and feet are facing away from each other and your leg bones are laterally rotated in the hip socket. All ballet dance is done in Turn Out, while modern dance often has movements that use the legs in Parallel. In Pilates, we do many exercises in Turn Out (see Pilates "V" from the Pilates Alphabet). Why Turn Out? Because it engages both the butt and inner thighs, and can help stabilize your pelvis during certain exercises.

PRONE

This term means lying on your belly.

THE POWERHOUSE

The Powerhouse is a term that came from Joe Pilates himself, used today mostly by New York trainers. The abdominals, butt, and inner thigh muscles, when working together, constitute the Powerhouse. This is where many of the Pilates exercises can be initiated. It is also the area that is challenged in many exercises. These muscles are the main stabilizing muscles of the body and are very important for preventing injury to the spine.

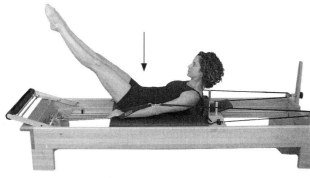

THE POWERHOUSE

RELEVÉ / HIGH HEEL FEET

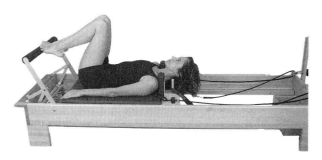

The foot is positioned so the weight of the foot is on the ball and toes. The ankle is in plantar flexion but the toes are in dorsiflexion.

SUPINE

This is a term that simply means lying on your back. Think: spine (Supine with the "u" taken out).

TORSO STABILITY

Torso Stability is accomplished mainly by abdominal strength and is one of the most important concepts in the Pilates Method. Most Pilates exercises require you to maintain a stable torso while the arms or legs move. Again, the abdominals are responsible for keeping the spine still while forces are moving around it. So when you are doing one of these Stability exercises (and you can tell if it is a Stability exercise if you hold the torso in one place for the duration of the exercise), simply think to yourself "don't move"—this is the essence of Stability.

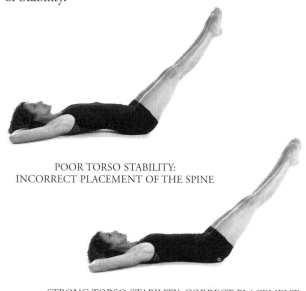

POOR TORSO STABILITY:
INCORRECT PLACEMENT OF THE SPINE

STRONG TORSO STABILITY: CORRECT PLACEMENT
OF THE SPINE—ABDOMINALS
KEEP BACK FLAT ON FLOOR

NEUTRAL SPINE, NEUTRAL PELVIS
WHAT'S IT ALL ABOUT, ELLIE?

Neutral Spine is one of the most subtle, yet powerful principles in the Pilates Alphabet. When the spine is neutral you have three spinal curves (cervical, thoracic, and lumbar) which function to absorb shock when running, jumping, or simply walking around town. And ultimately if you live in Neutral Spine, you will be putting the least amount of stress on the muscles and bones. That's the beauty of perfect posture: it actually feels better. We want to maintain and reinforce these natural curves and that is why we often work in Neutral Spine when performing stability exercises in Pilates.

Research has shown that the transverses abdominis (the deepest abdominal muscle) is more accessible when the pelvis is neutral. The transversus abdominis, with the help of the pelvic floor and multifidi (deep back muscles) form a triumvirate of stabilization for the spine. These deep stabilizers are key to healing spinal injuries and maintaining a healthy spine for life.

• FINDING NEUTRAL SPINE—NOT AS EASY AS YOU MIGHT THINK!

I spend the first two to three hours in my teacher trainings explaining and demonstrating how to find Neutral Spine with all the students. This is not a simple task, and it requires you to use your anatomy knowledge, proprioceptive skills and intuition as an instructor. Sorry, but there is no protocol here!

The first place to start is to find Neutral Pelvis, which is easily defined by objective measures: the ASIS (the hip bones) and the pubic bone form a triangle which forms a plane that should be parallel to the floor when lying down. You (or your client) can feel these bony landmarks with your fingers when supine, and this triangle of bones, when neutral, should create a flat table that could support a filled-to-the-brim double martini. When your pelvis is neutral, your martini will be perfectly balanced. If your pelvis is tilted forward (anterior pelvic tilt—arching your low back too much off the floor) or tilted back (posterior pelvic tilt—flattening your low back onto the floor), your martini will spill in one of those directions.

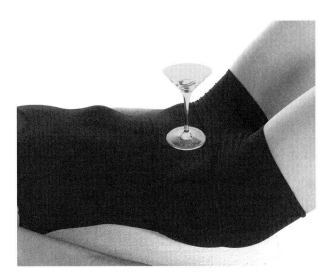

When lying supine in Neutral Pelvis you should have two areas that do not touch the floor beneath you: your neck and your low back (cervical and lumbar spine, respectively).

• NEUTRAL PELVIS VS. NEUTRAL SPINE

When lying supine, the spine does not act the same way as it does when standing, so you need to make adjustments accordingly.

Some people may find, when supine, that being in Neutral Pelvis puts their lumbar or thoracic spine into too much extension, and they will feel uncomfortable in this position. Why? Because even though their pelvis is neutral, their *spine* is not neutral—they have too much lumbar or thoracic curve and their back extensor muscles are contracted. This is not comfortable!

Neutral Spine cannot be measured objectively like Neutral Pelvis since everyone has different spinal curvatures, skeletal structures, and musculature. These put the spine into different positions when lying down. Even the size of someone's back side will change how the spine configures itself when supine. But as an instructor, your goal is to help your client find the optimal position of the spine and pelvis that allows the back muscles to remain relaxed while supine, while still maintaining some curvature.

• TOUCH YOUR CLIENTS

To help clients find Neutral Spine, trainers can put their hands underneath their client's lumbar spine to feel for too much space—your hand should not be able to slide all the way under the back to the other side. There should be a small space under the lumbar spine (not a huge one!). Also your hand should not be able to slide under their thoracic spine (ribcage). If you notice that the ribcage is lifted, cue your client to drop and release the ribcage down to the mat by engaging the upper abdominals. The thoracic spine should be making complete contact with the mat.

Trainers should also feel for contracted spinal extensor muscles—these muscles should stay relaxed. Ask your client if they feel comfortable—believe me, they'll know!

If necessary, tell the client to tilt the pelvis in the posterior direction, flattening their lumbar curve, to make the *spine* more neutral. For some, the pelvis needs to be slightly posterior for the spine to feel neutral and comfortable in the supine position. It is essential that the client feel comfortable when performing supine exercises, so if necessary, tuck them under a little. This is now *their Neutral* when lying down.

• SUPPORTED NEUTRAL

Neutral Spine can also be supported by placing a folded up towel or sticky mat underneath any portion of the spine that is unable to make contact with the mat. This is particularly good for people with anterior pelvic tilt or lordosis (who will need a towel under their lumbar spine), or people with convex thoracic curves (who will need a towel under their thoracic spine), or people with too much cervical curve (they will need support under their head to allow the neck to lengthen).

Supine Pilates stabilization exercises should never be performed with the spine unsupported (with too much extension), so make adjustments with each client individually so that they understand their Neutral Spine. Giving your client a proprioceptive tool under their back will help them to feel their abdominals engaging more and they will love you for it!

NEUTRAL SPINE VS. FLAT BACK

Many people from the New York school teach people to "tuck under" or flatten the curve of their low back when doing all supine Pilates exercises and when standing. In my method, I use Neutral Spine when it is safe and effective, and Flat Back when applicable.

My general rule of thumb is to use Neutral only when doing exercise that are "closed chain," meaning the legs are either on the floor *(Upper Abdominal Curl)*, or when using Pilates equipment, supported by a bar or straps *(Footwork*, Leg Series). Pilates Mat exercises are mostly "open chain," with the legs in the air, making the spine vulnerable to destabilization. In open chain exercises, it is safer to use the Flat Back position. Clients who have posterior pelvic tilt and/or very strong abdominals may experiment with bringing their pelvis more into a Neutral in open chain exercises. When on the equipment however, many exercises are closed chain, and it is an excellent opportunity to train your clients in Neutral Spine—working with the natural curves safely and effectively.

SPINAL FLEXION: WHAT YOU NEED TO KNOW

Spinal Flexion is one of the most common movements done in the Pilates Method.

FUNCTIONS

• Strengthens the abdominals

• Stretches the extensor muscles of the back

• Great for people with anterior pelvic tilt and lordosis (particularly lumbar flexion exercises)

GENERAL OBSTACLES

Like any movement, tightness in the oppositional muscle group will inhibit Range of Motion in the working muscle. With spinal flexion, the main movers are the abdominals and the opposing muscle groups are the back extensors. So if the back extensors are tight, in any portion of the spine, then it will be difficult to flex that part of the back.

For example, if someone has trouble coming up into an *Upper Abdominal Curl*, generally that points to a tightness in the neck and upper back. If someone has trouble imprinting their lower back onto the mat during a *Roll Down* or rolling exercise, then they probably have a tight lower back.

GENERAL CONTRAINDICATIONS

Because flexing the spine puts pressure and load onto the anterior structures of the spine; i.e. the intervertebra discs and bodies of the vertebrae, then any weakness or dysfunction of the anterior structures will make that person vulnerable to injury when flexing the spine. The more loaded the flexion, the more damaging. Please refer to the Loaded Flexion Continuum Chart (opposite page) for an overview of Pilates exercises and their concomitant load.

• DISC DYSFUNCTION

The intervertebral discs live in between the vertebral bodies of the spine and function as shock absorbers and cushioners for the huge amount of compression that loads the back every day. Most disc injuries are due to daily life activities that load the spine in flexion and ultimately weaken, herniate, or "slip" one or more discs. The following are the most common disc dysfunctions:

• Degeneration: Degeneration happens to all of us as we age, causing the disc to flatten due to the loss of its inner fluids. With too much degeneration, the cushioning action of the discs is lessened and inflammation and micro movements of the vertebral bodies that sandwich the discs can cause chronic pain.

• Herniation: A herniated disc is caused by the rupture of the cartilaginous outer layer which allows the inner fluid to escape into the spaces near the nerve roots along the spine—ouch!

• Subluxation: A disc can simply "slip" out of it's normal position and move anteriorly onto the nerve roots (double ouch!)—this is called subluxation.

In all these cases of disc dysfunction, loaded flexion would most likely be contraindicated and would greatly exacerbate any symptoms. Some disc problems are exacerbated by extension, but the majority can be relieved by extension.

• OSTEOPOROSIS

Osteoporosis is defined as a decrease in bone mass and bone density with an increased risk and/or incidence of fracture. Women over 50 should get checked to make sure they aren't suffering from osteoporosis or osteopenia (a less severe version). Flexion exercises are universally contraindicated for these conditions because it loads the vertebral bodies which are weakened and vulnerable to breakage. Instead, do exercises where the spine is in neutral or extension.

LOADED FLEXION CONTINUUM

LEAST LOADED	SEMI LOADED	VERY LOADED!

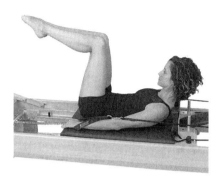 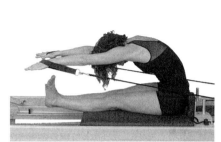 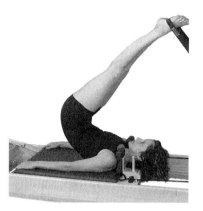

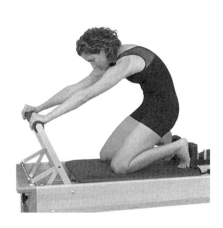 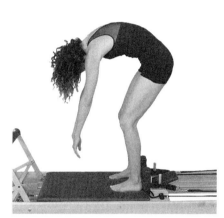 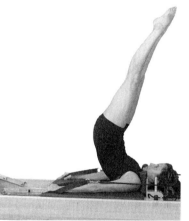

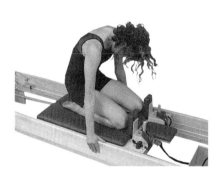 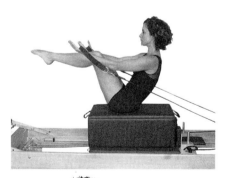 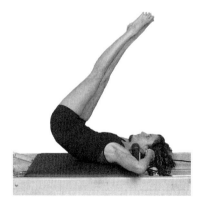

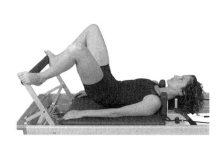 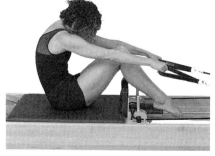 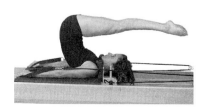

SPINAL EXTENSION: WHAT YOU NEED TO KNOW

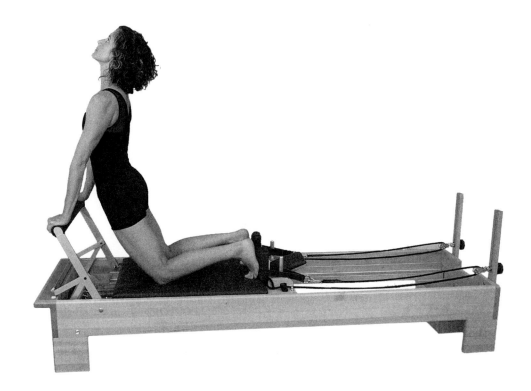

Back extension exercises are normally performed prone (on your belly), and actively use your spinal extensors. In many Mat exercise, spinal extension originates from the head and neck and sequences through the spine to the upper back and finally the lower back.

FUNCTIONS

• Strengthens the spine and neck extensors

• Stretches the front body; namely the abdominals and chest

• Great for people with posterior pelvic tilt; who generally present with lengthened lumbar extensors and tight abdominals. For these people, it is not as essential to initiate full back extension with the hip extensors since they are already living in a relatively "tucked" position

• Great for people with kyphosis (particularly upper back extension exercises)

DISC DYSFUNCTION

Extension of the spine can be indicated for people suffering from vertebral disc dysfunction (herniated, bulging or subluxated disc) because it opens the space between the vertebral bodies anteriorly and allows the disc to return to its proper space, away from the spinal nerve roots which, when impinged, cause pain. All spinal extension exercises are great for kyphotic people (particularly upper back extension) who have lengthened upper back extensors.

CAUTION

Be mindful when training people with lordosis and anterior pelvic tilt since those individuals will have short/tight lumbar extensors and hip flexors along with weak/lengthened abdominals and hip extensors (glutes and hamstrings). They should only do the *Cygnet* (baby *Swan*), lifting only their head, neck, and upper back, keeping their lower back stable; using the Abdominal Scoop and hip extensors (glutes and hamstrings) to stabilize the pelvis. This should feel like a butt and hamstring exercise for these people; not a lower back exercise.

THE ROLE OF HIP EXTENSORS

Back Extension and Hip Extension flow together since the base of the spine (Sacrum) is shared and continuous with the hips and pelvis. Full back extension (think: *High Swan*), cannot be fully achieved without the hip extension.

Spinal Extension should be initiated by hip extensors and abdominals to protect the lower back from hyperextension and to allow full spinal extension. This means starting every time with scooping the belly in and tucking your pelvis under with your glutes and hamstrings.

People with weakness in their hip extensors (glutes and hamstrings) will not be able to do full back extension in a prone position because the pelvis cannot stabilize on the mat and the spine will not be able to fully lift off the mat. This issue is often coupled with/caused by tight hip flexors.

GENERAL CONTRAINDICATIONS

Because extending the spine puts pressure and load onto the posterior structures of the spine; i.e. the tranverse foramen (where the spinal nerves come out) and the facet joints, then any weakness or dysfunction of the posterior structures will make that person vulnerable to injury when extending the spine. The more loaded the extension, the more damaging.

• STENOSIS AND FACET JOINT PROBLEMS

Spinal Stenosis is the narrowing of the lumbar spinal canal, an arthritic process, which happens as a normal part of aging. People with this problem will experience minor to severe nerve impingement.

Facet joints are in almost constant motion with the spine and simply wear out and/or degenerate in people as they age. When facet joints become worn there may be a reaction of the bone of the joint underneath producing bone spurs and an enlargement of the joints

(osteoarthritis). This condition may also be referred to as "facet joint disease" or "facet joint syndrome" and can be quite painful for people when they move their spine. In both the case of stenosis and facet joint problems, extension will exacerbate symptoms and flexion and/or Neutral Spine may alleviate them.

• OSTEOPOROSIS AND STENOSIS

Three words: Neutral, Neutral and Neutral.

THE ROLE OF ABDOMINALS

Scooping the abdominals in toward the spine while attempting spinal extension will help to distribute the extension throughout the spine. When abdominals are not engaged, most of the back extension will occur at L2-3.

Thus, it is essential when doing prone full back extension exercises to initiate the movement with both the abdominals and hip extensors. I always cue "scoop your belly in toward your spine, squeeze your glutes and tuck your pelvis under, and then rise up into back extension."

ASSISTING PEOPLE

When teaching prone back extension exercises to folks with weak abdominals, glutes and hamstrings, I recommend assisting them to prevent compression in their lumbar spines. Hold their calves down (or you can strap their legs down if you have access to a Cadilllac) so they can stabilize their pelvis and activate their glutes and hamstrings. This will enable them to rise all the way up into a full *Swan*. Try it—you'll see them rise like a phoenix from the ashes.

HOW TO CREATE AN HOUR-LONG SESSION

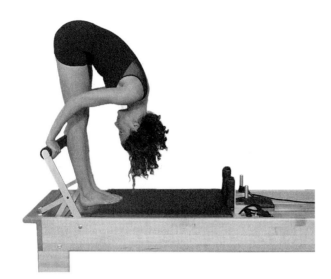

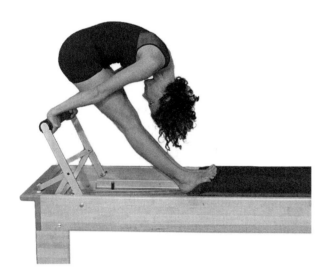

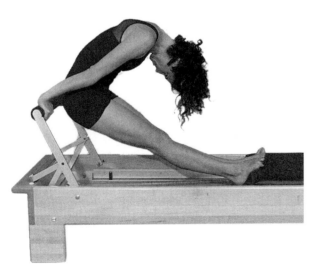

Think of the repertoire as your palette, from which you, the Pilates artist, should pick and choose based on your knowledge of what you or your client needs.

When planning a session for your client, make sure that you:

1. WARM UP

Footwork and the Supine Series is an excellent warm up. I never skip any of these exercises when I am teaching the Reformer.

2. WORK ALL PARTS OF THE BODY

Core: We can break down core exercises into **stabilization** and **articulation** exercises. It is important to do both kinds of core strengthening, but equally important to notice if your client needs more of one than the other. For instance, if you are training a very stiff, tight client whose spine barely moves in any direction, then articulation exercises will be preferable to stabilization exercises. And conversely, if you have a noodle-y client who is hyper-mobile and can't keep her trunk still to save her life, then stabilization would make more sense for her.

*Rehabilitation Note: When working with clients who have spinal injuries, especially disc dysfunction, stabilization is the preferred core strengthening technique. Spinal flexion, extension, and/or rotation may exacerbate certain back injuries.

Core Stabilization:
Exercises: *Hundred, Coordination, Leg Series, Kneeling Series, all Flat Back exercises*

Core Articulation:
Exercises: *Mermaid, all Roll Down exercises, Teasers*

Lower Body:
Exercises: *Footwork, Jumping, Splits, Hamstrings, Leg Series*

Upper Body:
Exercises: *Arm Series (Supine, Prone, Kneeling, Side)*

Total Body:
Exercises: *Tendon Stretch, Plank Series, Twist, Snake, Star*

3. MOVE THE SPINE IN ALL DIRECTIONS

Flexion: Generally we start the workout with flexion exercises because it fires up our abdominals and warms up the spine.
Exercises: *The Hundred, Overhead, Short and Long Spine Stretch, all Round Back exercises*

Extension: After doing a series of flexion exercises, make sure to do spinal extension exercises to balance the spine.
Exercises: *Pulling the Ropes, Rocking Swan, Breaststroke, Down Stretch*

Side Bending or Lateral Flexion: Side bending stretches out the abdominal obliques and quadratus lumborum and can help lateral imbalances like scoliosis.
Exercises: *Mermaid, Side Sit Ups, Up & Over a Barrel*

Twisting or Spinal Rotation: Twisting is healthy for the spine, but it is not indicated for disc dysfunction.
Exercises: *Twist, Twist with Stick, Stomach Massage: Bouquet, Mermaid: Carve a Sphere*

4. LET THE SESSION FLOW

Choose an exercise order that makes sense for flow so that you don't have to change the springs with each exercise and so your client is not getting up and off the machine every minute.

5. USE MORE THAN ONE PIECE OF EQUIPMENT IF POSSIBLE

Mat work really focuses on the abs. Wunda Chair has some killer upper body and leg conditioning exercises. Springboard challenges stability, strength and coordination. Cadillac is great for rehab and focusing on specific problem areas.

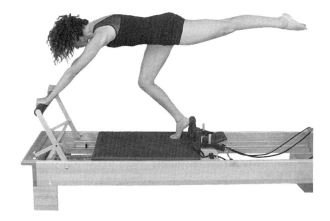

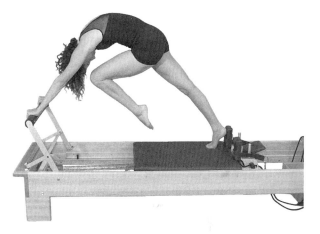

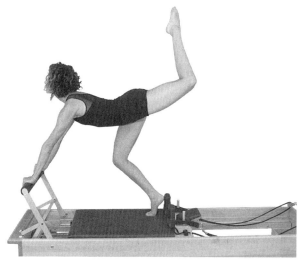

HOW TO USE THIS MANUAL

The manual has what I consider to be a complete repertoire of Reformer Exercises; some are classic Pilates, while others are invented by myself or other trainers over the years.

THE LEVELS

We have broken down the levels into:
• **Beginning**
• **Intermediate**
• **Advanced**
• **Super Advanced**

THE SERIES

In the Pilates Method, the Reformer and the Mat are taught as series, meaning each level has a specific order and flow. (Exercises on the Cadillac, Chair, and Barrel are not generally taught in a series; they are discrete and can be added in to a workout to address specific issues you or your client may have.)

When teaching a client in a one-hour time frame, you will have to use your best judgment when deciding what is essential for that client. You will probably not be able to do all the exercises in a given level in one hour. (Even the beginning series can be quite long!) The series is really a way to organize the exercises on the equipment, giving you a framework and an order.

Beginning Series: Start at the beginning of the manual and go in order, doing all of the beginning exercises.

Intermediate Series: Start at the beginning of the manual and do the essential beginning and all the intermediate exercises in order. Any exercises that have a beginning version and an intermediate version, replace with the more advanced version and omit the easier one (i.e., *Chest Expansion* is done sitting on the long box in the beginning series but kneeling in the intermediate series).

Advanced and Super Advanced Series: Start at the beginning of the manual and do all the beginning and intermediate exercises and selected advanced and super advanced exercises in order. For any exercise that has both an intermediate and an advanced version, do the more advanced version and omit the easier one (i.e., *Reverse Teaser* can be replaced with *Teaser* on the long box).

Remember, the levels of the exercises are meant to help you learn the Pilates Method in a natural progression for your body. Most importantly, the levels are meant to help you not hurt yourself. The intermediate and advanced exercises require a fair amount of core strength to perform properly. You could injure yourself or your client if you try to push beyond the appropriate level.

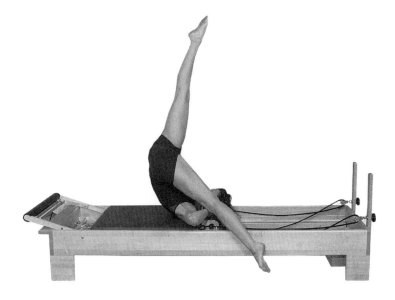

OTHER HELPFUL THINGS

Please read the **cues** and **obstacles sections** for each exercise carefully to make sure you understand the correct form.

As a teacher, "do no harm" is your most important mantra! So read the **contraindications** carefully to make sure you're not hurting yourself or anyone else.

Specific Modifications are outlined in each exercise if there are any. They are meant to help you advance at your own pace. If you or your client feel strain in your low back or neck at anytime, or if the exercise is just too difficult, please do not continue with the movement; look for modifications instead.

GENERAL MODIFICATIONS

When learning new exercises it is common for certain aches and pains to develop. The following are a few common problems that people face when they are still in the process of gaining strength and stability. Please read through this section even if you don't have any of these problems yet. The point is to prevent potential overuse or strain of your muscles and tissues.

How to modify to protect the low back:
In general, if you suffer from low back pain, you need to know a few tips to keep you from further contributing to your problems. Always modify any exercise that requires you to support your legs out in front of you while keeping your belly scooped or your back flat on the mat. Experiment with the following modifications:

• Bend your knees if the exercise requires straight legs.

• Keep your legs high enough so that you can absolutely maintain a scooped belly and a flat back on the mat.

• Stop if you feel back strain.

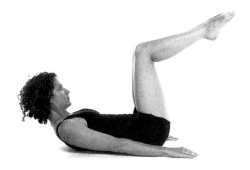

PROTECT YOUR LOW BACK: BEGINNING

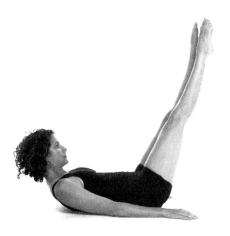

PROTECT YOUR LOW BACK: INTERMEDIATE

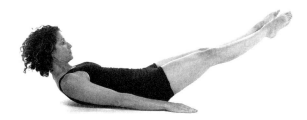

PROTECT YOUR LOW BACK: ADVANCED

How to avoid wrist compression when up on your arms:

- Put your hand as far forward on the bar as possible to lessen wrist extension. Think of putting the heel of the hand on the bar and fingers reaching down toward the floor.

- Keep your shoulders properly aligned. Think of rolling the shoulder blades down away from the ears so you are supporting your body weight from the back muscles.

- Think of pressing away from the bar with your back strength.

- Don't let your weight bear down into the wrist; instead, press away from gravity.

- Don't hyperextend your elbows: keep the inner elbow creases facing each other.

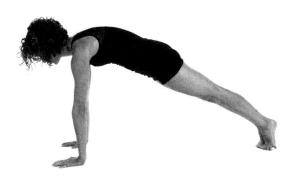

PROTECT YOUR WRISTS: CORRECT—LIFT UP FROM THE WRISTS AND SHOULDERS AND SOFTEN THE ELBOWS

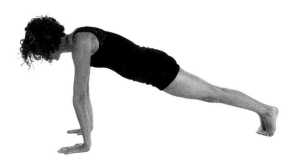

PROTECT YOUR WRISTS: INCORRECT—AVOID DROPPING INTO YOUR WRISTS, ELBOWS, AND SHOULDERS

How to do a rolling exercise: Never onto your neck!

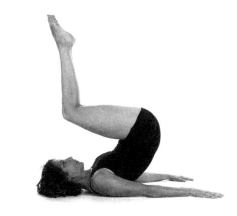

CORRECT NECK PLACEMENT: BALANCE BETWEEN YOUR SHOULDER BLADES ON YOUR "THORACIC SHELF"

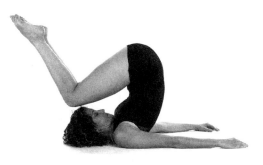

INCORRECT NECK PLACEMENT: DON'T ROLL ONTO YOUR NECK

There are several exercises on the Reformer that require you to roll onto your upper back (*Short Spine Stretch, Overhead,* etc.).

- Do not roll onto your neck; instead, stop and balance between your shoulder blades.

- Use control when rolling back. Don't roll back so fast that you can't control your momentum.

- Scoop your abdominals in to help stop yourself from rolling back too far.

EXERCISES

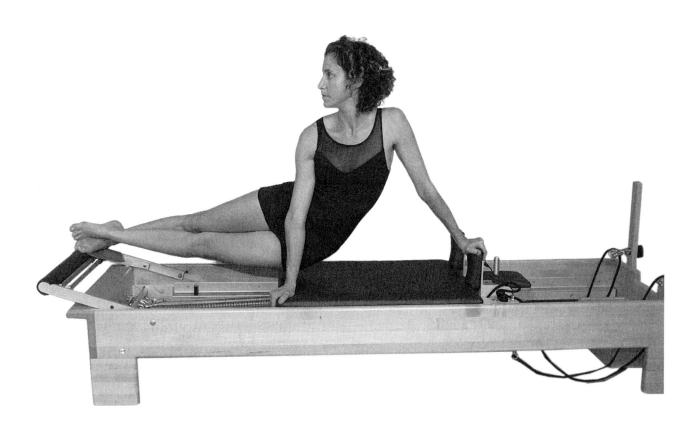

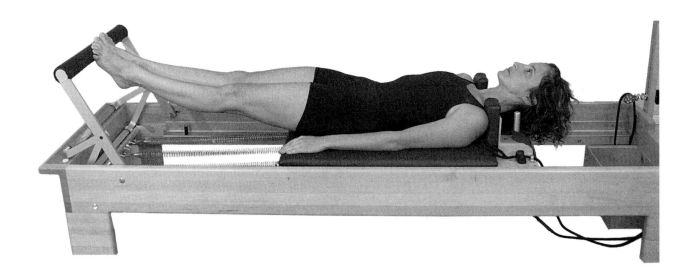

Footwork is the first series of exercises done on the Reformer. It uses the large muscles of the legs to "warm-up" the body, plus it's a great opportunity to reinforce the concept of Neutral Spine.

WHICH VARIATIONS SHOULD YOU DO?

The variations can be added in to a workout program to address the individual's needs. For instance, a person with postural bowlegs will benefit from additional external rotation *Footwork (Heels in First Position, Heels in Second Position)*. A person with ankle instability will benefit from *Toes in Parallel* and *Combo*. *Internal Rotation* has been recently added to the repertoire to balance all the external rotation done in Pilates and dance; the hip joint needs to be used in all ROM for long-term health. Single leg variations are great for knee, hip and ankle rehabilitation, or simply for correcting imbalances.

FOOTBAR SETTING: HIGH VS. LOW

• Use high bar if client is short or has an anterior pelvic tilt. High bar is the default position.

• Use low bar if client is very tall, has tight hips and/or cannot achieve Neutral Spine with high bar. Low bar works the back of the legs a bit more and challenges the abdominals as you straighten the legs.

• For very tall and/or inflexible clients: move carriage away from home so that the client is not in too deep of knee and hip flexion.

FOOTWORK ON THE JUMPBOARD

The Jumpboard is a fantastic functional tool to use for Footwork since it replicates standing and walking on the ground more than the Footbar. It is also a great diagnostic tool for teachers to see their clients alignment issues at the level of the hip, knee and ankle. And finally, Footwork on the Jumpboard is the best warm up for the feet and ankles to prepare a client for Jumping. See the Jumping Prep/Footwork page (page 182), for specific positions and descriptions of Footwork on the Jumpboard.

PROPS

A small squishy ball is great between the knees for the parallel positions to cue the inner thighs. Clients with postural knock knees (hyper extended knees with lateral rotation of the femurs) will benefit from having a larger ball between their ankles, to cue the long adductor and allow space for them to straighten the legs without knocking. Client's with postural bowlegs (hyperextended knees with medial rotation of the femurs) will benefit from having a theraband tied around the lower thighs to cue proper knee alignment. Do not put a ball between the knees of someone with internal rotation since it will exacerbate this condition.

FIRST GEAR VS. SECOND GEAR

First gear pulls the springs into "pre-load," which makes the exercise more challenging for the leg muscles, and is great for healthy clients who need conditioning. Second gear has no "pre-load," which challenges the cores muscles and hamstrings more, especially when returning the carriage to its home position. Second gear is the preferred setting for client's with lower limb injuries, because the joints (hip, knee, ankle) will not be as stressed on the initiation of the movement. I tend to use first gear because it is simply more resistance—and I like to really strengthen my legs.

HEAD REST SETTING: UP OR DOWN?

The classic setting for *Footwork* is head rest up, because it facilitates abdominal engagement and ribcage stability when the head is up slightly. If your client has tension in their neck when the head rest is up, then try putting it down. Ask the client their preference, and use your judgement about which position is appropriate.

THE CLASSIC 4 FOOTWORK POSITIONS

1. *First Position*
2. *Monkey on a Branch*
3. *Heels in Parallel*
4. *Calf Raises*

FOOTWORK VARIATIONS

Heels in First Position/Second Position
Toes in Parallel
Internal Rotation
Combo
Single Leg on Heel/Toe
Sleeper
Ballet Combo

SPRING SETTINGS

Start everyone with light resistance to cue the core muscles and the hamstrings, and then increase resistance to challenge client's lower limb strength. Injured clients, and those with overdeveloped quadriceps will benefit from doing *Footwork* on lighter resistance (2–3 springs). Larger, stronger clients can use heavier resistance (3–4 heavy springs).

ALIGNMENT CUES FOR ALL FOOTWORK

- Keep pelvis neutral (it is very easy to tuck to initiate the movement).

- Do not allow ribs to "pop" up and destabilize the torso.

- Work both legs evenly (look for one knee straightening before the other).

- Do not hyperextend or lock knees when straightening legs—pull inner thighs together.

- Think: extend from the hip instead of the knees. This will engage the hamstrings and lessen the work of the quads.

- Keep neck, jaw and shoulders relaxed.

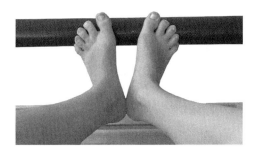

MACHINE SET UP

- springs: 2 red & 1 blue, 3 red, or more...
- bar: high or low
- ropes: N/A
- risers: N/A
- headrest: up or down

FUNCTIONS & TARGET MUSCLES

- Warms up body
- Strengthens quads, hamstrings, hip adductors, and hip external rotators
- Teaches pelvic stabilization and disassociation of femur from pelvis
- External rotation *Footwork* is great for clients with postural bowlegs (femurs medially rotated and knees hyper-extended)

ALIGNMENT CUES & OBSTACLES

- Do not over rotate at ankle or hip, keep knees no wider than carriage
- Feel low glutes working on push and helping to control the carriage home
- Feel inner thighs reach toward one another to straighten legs
- Do not lower heels while pushing carriage out
- To cue hamstrings, pull sit bones together on the way out, and pull in from the hamstrings to bring the carriage home—think: 50% hamstrings, 50% quads

VARIATIONS & PEEL BACKS

- For clients with knock knees, where the knees knock before full extension, place a ball or something squishy between the heels/ankles to enable the legs to straighten fully
- Use light springs for people with over-developed quads to cue into hamstrings and abdominals
- **Variation:** *Heels in First Position:* Place heels on the bar with feet in Pilates "V" with heels together and toes apart, externally rotating at the hip. Focus on heel to sit bones connection to cue the hamstrings
- **Variation:** *Heels in Second Position:* Place heels on outside edges of footbar with hips in external rotation—like 2nd position in ballet. Do not splay knees open, keep inner thighs engaged. In this position it easy to hyperextend lumbar spine while straightening the knees, so focus on low abdominals stabilizing top of sacrum

IMAGINE...a lead blanket, like the ones used during X-rays, is draped over your torso, keeping the rib cage relaxed and heavy.

ELLIE SAYS..."Crease at the hips to bring carriage home—don't tuck."

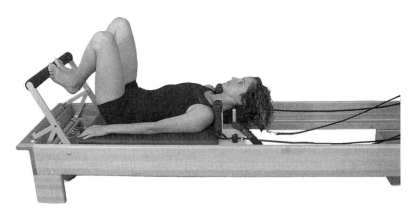

1. Starting Position—*10 repetitions each position*
Lying on back with head on headrest, place toes on the bar with feet in Pilates "V" with heels together and toes apart.

Inhale to prepare

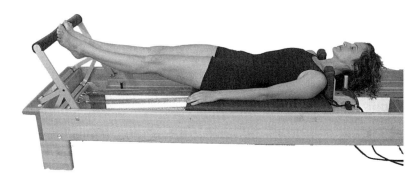

2. Exhale
Feel abdominals engage and push carriage out straightening the knees and pulling inner thighs together. Maintain Neutral Spine and Pelvis.

3. Inhale
Bend knees and control carriage back to Starting Position without coming all the way home between repetitions—do not slam the carriage into home.

VARIATIONS:

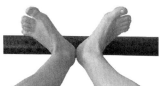

Heels in First

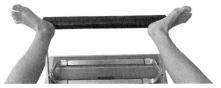

Heels in Second

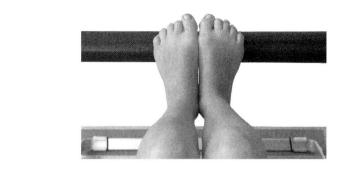

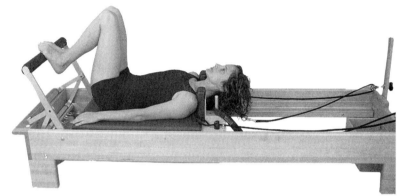

MACHINE SET UP
- springs: 2 red & 1 blue, or 3 red, or more...
- bar: high or low
- ropes: N/A
- risers: N/A
- headrest: up or down

FUNCTIONS & TARGET MUSCLES
- Warms up body
- Strengthens quads, hamstrings and intrinsic muscles of the foot
- Teaches pelvic stabilization and disassociation of femur from pelvis
- Great exercise for clients with weak arches, weak ankles, flat feet, and rigid feet

ALIGNMENT CUES & OBSTACLES
- Focus on hamstrings pulling carriage home—think: heel-hamstring connection
- Imagine you're making a C-Curve with your foot—pointing your toes while flexing your heels. But keep foot lengthened and relaxed—don't cramp your feet!
- Pull medial ankles together to cue inner thighs

VARIATIONS & PEEL BACKS
- Use light springs for people with overdeveloped quads to cue hamstrings and abdominals
- Put a small squishy ball or something small between the knees to reinforce the inner thigh connection
- For clients with knock knees, where the knees knock before full extension, place a ball between the heels/ankles to enable the legs to straighten fully
- For clients with bow legs, where the knees do not stay together when legs straighten, put a theraband around the lower thighs/knees to cue proper alignment
- **Variation:** To really cue the hamstrings, try pulsing the carriage in, coming almost home and going out only a few inches, accenting the "in" direction

IMAGINE...*you are a bird on a perch.*

ELLIE SAYS...*"Yummy foot massage!"*

1. Starting Position—*10 repetitions*
Lying on back with head on headrest, place your feet on the bar just below the ball of your foot (at the high part of the arch), and wrap toes around bar keeping toes long with ankles, knees, and inner thighs squeezing together. Find the place on your foot where you feel "maximum wrappage," so that your foot really wraps around the bar.

Inhale to prepare

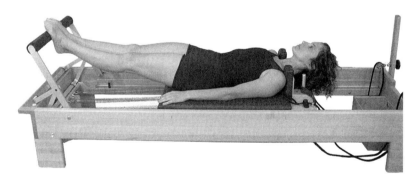

2. Exhale
Feel abdominals engage and push carriage out, straightening the knees—feel VMO (medial quad) working. Maintain Neutral Spine and Pelvis.

3. Inhale
Bend knees and control carriage back to Starting Position without coming all the way home between repetitions—do not slam the carriage into home.

HEELS IN PARALLEL

MACHINE SET UP
- springs: 2 red & 1 blue, or 3 red, or more...
- bar: high or low
- ropes: N/A
- risers: N/A
- headrest: up or down

FUNCTIONS & TARGET MUSCLES
- Warms up body
- Strengthens quads, hamstrings, and dorsiflexors
- Teaches pelvic stabilization and disassociation of femur from pelvis
- Great exercise for clients who wear high heels

ALIGNMENT CUES & OBSTACLES
- Best *Footwork* exercise to cue the hamstrings—think: heel-hamstring connection
- To help client feel hamstring engagement, place your hands under your client's heels and have them press down onto your hands as they press the carriage away
- Really flex your feet and pull your toes back
- Reach big toe metatarsal forward and pull pinky toes back to cue inner thighs and peroneals and to correct ankle supination

VARIATIONS & PEEL BACKS
- Use light springs for people with over-developed quads to cue into hamstrings and abdominals
- Put a small squishy ball or something small between the knees to reinforce the inner thigh connection
- For clients with knock knees, where the knees knock before full extension, place a ball or squishy thing between the heels/ankles to enable the legs to straighten fully
- For clients with bow legs, where the knees do not stay together when they straighten their legs, put a theraband around lower thighs/knees to cue proper knee alignment
- Can also work with heels in line with sit bones in a more natural parallel—feel free to place balls between knees and/or ankles so client can feel alignment

IMAGINE... *you are standing on a floor.*

ELLIE SAYS... *"This is the most stable of all Footwork exercises, and the best way to see your client's leg alignment issues."*

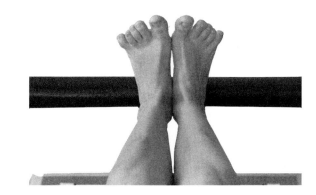

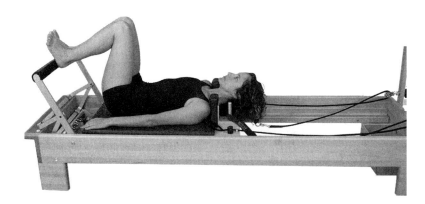

1. Starting Position—*10 repetitions*
Lying on back with head on headrest, place heels on bar with flexed feet—ankles, knees, and inner thighs touching.

Inhale to prepare

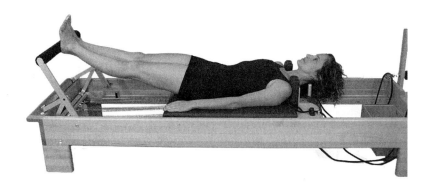

2. Exhale
Feel abdominals engage and press heels gently down as you push carriage out, straightening the knees—feel VMO (medial quad) working as you fully extend. Maintain Neutral Spine.

3. Inhale
Bend knees and control carriage back to Starting Position without coming all the way home between repetitions—do not slam the carriage into home.

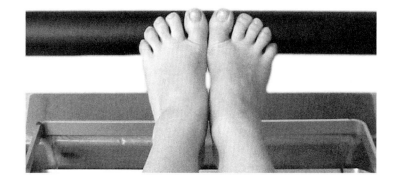

MACHINE SET UP
- springs: 2 red & 1 blue, or 3 red, or more...
- bar: high or low
- ropes: N/A
- risers: N/A
- headrest: up or down

FUNCTIONS & TARGET MUSCLES
- Warms up body
- Strengthens quads, hamstrings, ankles, and feet
- Teaches pelvic stabilization and disassociation of femur from pelvis

ALIGNMENT CUES & OBSTACLES
- Do not drop heels while pushing out
- I've heard people call this position "Barbie feet"
- Do not allow hips to internally rotate when knees straighten
- Feel the big toe metatarsal-VMO connection

VARIATIONS & PEEL BACKS
- Use light springs for people with overdeveloped quads to cue into hamstrings and abdominals
- Put a small squishy ball or something small between the knees to reinforce the inner thigh and VMO connection
- Pull medial ankles together to cue inner thighs
- For clients with knock knees, where the knees knock before full extension, place a ball or something squishy between the heels/ankles to enable the legs to straighten fully
- For clients with bow legs, where the knees do not stay together when they straighten their legs, put a bigger ball or something squishy between the knees to keep inner thigh connection and proper alignment
- Can also work with heels in line with sit bones in a more natural parallel—feel free to place balls between knees and/or ankles so client can feel alignment

IMAGINE...*you are a Barbie.*

ELLIE SAYS...*"Great to strengthen the VMO and the ankles."*

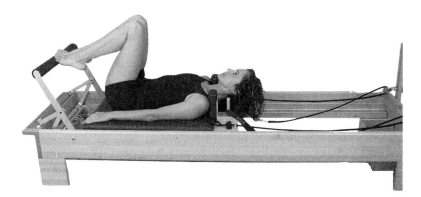

1. Starting Position—*10 repetitions*
Lying on back with head on headrest, place toes on bar with heels lifted (similar to relevé in dance)—ankles, knees, and inner thighs touching.

Inhale to prepare

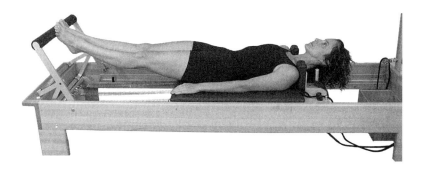

2. Exhale
Feel abdominals engage and push carriage out, straightening the knees—feel VMO (medial quad) working. Maintain Neutral Spine and Pelvis.

3. Inhale
Bend knees and control carriage back to Starting Position without coming all the way home between repetitions—do not slam the carriage into home.

INTERNAL ROTATION *footwork series*

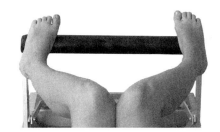

MACHINE SET UP
- springs: 2 red & 1 blue, or 3 red, or more...
- bar: high or low
- ropes: N/A
- risers: N/A
- headrest: up or down

FUNCTIONS & TARGET MUSCLES
- Warms up body
- Strengthens quads, works hamstrings, and internal rotators of the hip
- Teaches pelvic stabilization and disassociation of femur from pelvis
- Great for postural knock knees (lateral rotation of femurs with hyperextension of knees)

ALIGNMENT CUES & OBSTACLES
- Legs should be far enough apart so knees do not knock when straightening the legs
- Make sure the rotation occurs at hip joint and not knees or ankles
- Keep feet flexed to ensure proper ankle/foot alignment—do not sickle feet
- Important for ballet and modern dancers to balance excessive external rotation
- Clients with slim hips should narrow their stance—don't force excessive internal rotation

VARIATIONS & PEEL BACKS
- **Variation:** *VMO Pulses:* Only press out as far as you can while still keeping knees glued together (about halfway out). Pulse the carriage in and out, accenting the "in", always keeping knees squeezing together. You should feel the burn in your VMO (Vastus Medialis Obliquus, oblique fibers of the medial quadriceps, just above the knee). VMO strengthening is important for knee rehabilitation

IMAGINE...*you are the antithesis of a ballet dancer.*

ELLIE SAYS...*"It is important for hip health to work the legs in all ROM of the hip joint. Also, internal rotation is a part of normal gait sequencing."*

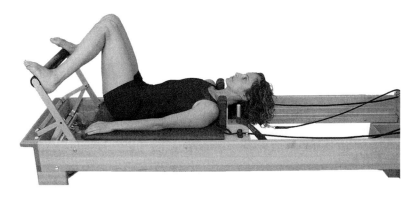

1. Starting Position—*10 repetitions*
Lying on back with head on headrest, place arches on bar slightly wider than hips, and roll femurs toward one another creating internal rotation at the hip, bringing knees together.

Inhale to prepare

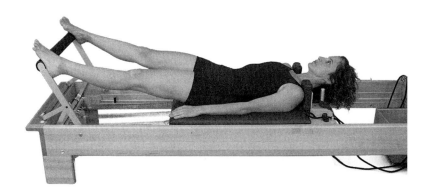

2. Exhale
Feel abdominals engage and push carriage out, straightening the legs (the knees will naturally separate). Maintain Neutral Spine and Pelvis.

3. Inhale
Bend knees and control carriage back to Starting Position without coming all the way home between repetitions—do not slam the carriage into home.

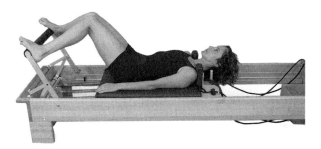

VARIATION: VMO Pulses

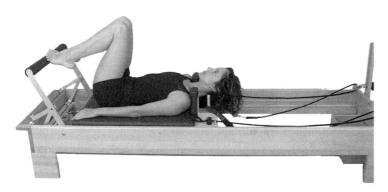

1. Starting Position—*10 repetitions*
Place toes on bar with heels high (similar to relevé in dance)—ankles, knees, and inner thighs touching.

Inhale to prepare

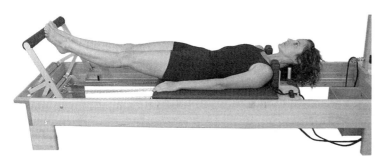

2. Exhale
Stabilize pelvis and spine with abdominals and push carriage out until legs are straight, keeping heels high.

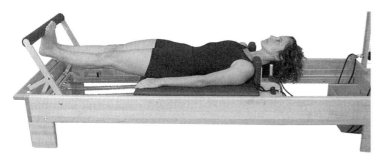

3. Inhale
Take 3 counts to slowly lower heels, maintaining straight and parallel legs, keeping weight on all 5 metatarsals.

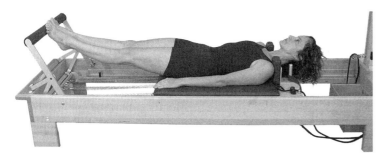

4. Exhale
Take 3 counts to slowly raise heels.

Repeat *Calf Raises* 10 times and return to Starting Position.

MACHINE SET UP
- springs: 2 red & 1 blue, or 3 red
- bar: high or low
- ropes: N/A
- risers: N/A
- headrest: up or down

FUNCTIONS & TARGET MUSCLES
- Strengthens and stretches plantar flexors
- Teaches ankle stability—great for ankle rehabilitation

ALIGNMENT CUES & OBSTACLES
- Do not allow hips to internally rotate when lowering heels—even though legs are parallel the low glutes/lateral hip rotators need to work
- Do not tuck pelvis while raising heels—keep quads relaxed and really just work calves
- Keep ankles stable in plantar flexion by keeping weight equally distributed between big toe and pinky toe
- The movement should be smooth, slow and sustained—don't drop the ankles down
- Keep even weight on all metatarsals

IMAGINE...*you are slowly dropping your heels into mud.*

ELLIE SAYS...*"This exercise is a great example of the beauty of the Reformer. Where else can you take the ankle through its full Range of Motion, strengthening and stretching while lying supine, and keeping perfect alignment?"*

MACHINE SET UP
- springs: 2 red & 1 blue, or 3 red
- bar: high or low
- ropes: N/A
- risers: N/A
- headrest: up or down

FUNCTIONS & TARGET MUSCLES
- Strengthens and stretches plantar flexors
- Works quads and hamstrings
- Teaches ankle stability—great for ankle rehabilitation

ALIGNMENT CUES & OBSTACLES
- Do not allow hips to internally rotate when lowering heels—even though legs are parallel, the low glutes/lateral hip rotators need to work
- Do not tuck pelvis while raising heels—keep quads relaxed and really just work calves
- Keep ankles stable in plantar flexion by keeping weight equally distributed between big toe and pinky toe
- Perform the ankle motion quickly, accentuating the "up" motion of the heels, but don't jam into ankles—keep the movement fluid

IMAGINE...*you are dropping your heels into fire—once they descend, you must lift them up—but quick!*

ELLIE SAYS...*"This one has rhythm—adding percussiveness to your ankle work."*

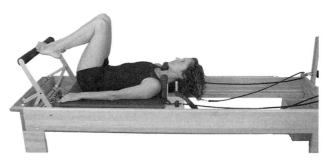

1. Starting Position—*10 repetitions*
Place toes on bar with heels high (similar to relevé in dance) with ankles, knees, and inner thighs touching.

Inhale to prepare

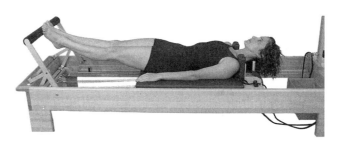

2. Exhale
Stabilize pelvis and spine with abdominals and push carriage out until legs are straight, keeping heels high.

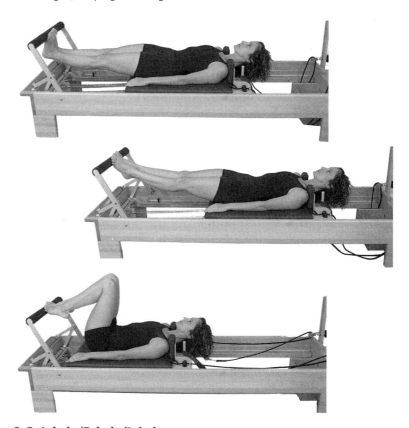

3–5. Inhale/Exhale/Inhale
Lower heels under the bar. Raise the heels and accent the "up." Bend knees and return carriage almost all the way to home, then repeat sequence.

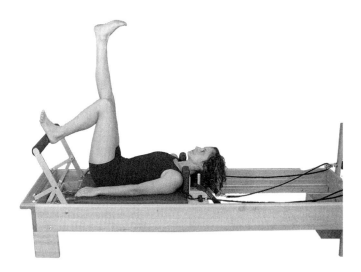

1. Starting Position—*10 repetitions*

Lying on back with head on the headrest and legs in parallel, place heel of one foot on the bar. Hold opposite leg in Table Top position, or straight up to the sky, with arms resting by sides.

Inhale to prepare

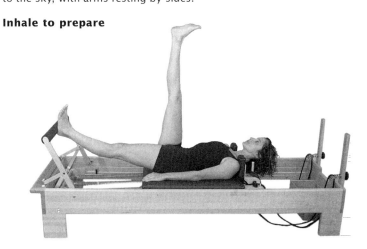

2. Exhale

Feel abdominals engage and push carriage out, straightening knee—feel VMO (medial quad) working. Maintain Neutral Spine and Pelvis.

3. Inhale

Bend knee and control carriage back to Starting Position without coming all the way home between repetitions—do not slam the carriage into home.

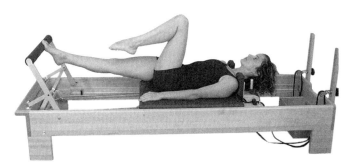

VARIATION: On Toe

MACHINE SET UP
- springs: 2 red
- bar: high or low
- ropes: N/A
- risers: N/A
- headrest: up or down

FUNCTIONS & TARGET MUSCLES
- Strengthens quads and hamstrings one leg at a time (great for rehab)
- Works internal obliques and multifidi

ALIGNMENT CUES & OBSTACLES
- Do not allow pelvis to rotate—feel internal oblique of working leg stabilizing pelvis

VARIATIONS & PEEL BACKS
- **Variation:** To increase work of low abdominals, keep nonworking leg under footbar as you come home
- **Variation:** To challenge client's coordination: start with nonworking leg extended over bar, as working leg straightens, bend nonworking leg into Table Top position. Reverse the action as carriage moves toward home—working leg bends and nonworking leg straightens reaching over footbar
- **Variation:** On Toe (high relevé) to challenge ankle stability

IMAGINE...*you are standing on one leg while keeping your pelvis stable.*

ELLIE SAYS...*"These exercises are key for knee rehab."*

MACHINE SET UP

- springs: 2 red
- bar: high or low
- ropes: N/A
- risers: N/A
- headrest: up

FUNCTIONS & TARGET MUSCLES

- Strengthens upper hamstrings and low glutes
- Works glute meds, quads, abdominals, and rotators in turn out
- Teaches side lying neutral

ALIGNMENT CUES & OBSTACLES

- Keep spine in a straight line with pelvis directly under skull
- Maintain side lying neutral with waist lifted and hips stacked
- Use pillow on head rest if client has neck issues or tension
- Do not tuck pelvis—stick the booty out
- Really flex the working foot and press into heel to fire the low glutes/hamstrings

IMAGINE...*you are pushing out from the upper hamstring.*

ELLIE SAYS...*"Your clients will fall asleep if you do this when they don't need it!"*

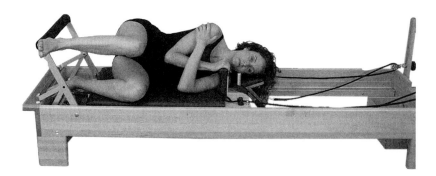

1. Starting Position—*10 to 20 repetitions*
Lie on side placing head on head rest and heel of top leg at the front corner of the bar. Bottom leg is bent and resting on carriage.

Inhale to prepare

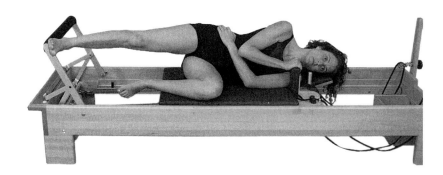

2. Exhale
Extend leg, cuing into the hamstring and low glute. Keep pelvis square. Keep top leg parallel to floor.

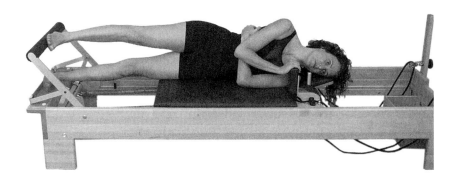

VARIATION: Hip Hike

Variation: *Hip Hike*: Use low bar and align your legs straight with your torso. Straighten top leg and press carriage out. Allow the top hip to hike. Then press the hip away from ribcage, engaging gluteus medius. Hold this lengthened position. Repeat 10 times. This variation is excellent for people with unilateral gluteus medius weakness which results in "hip hiking" on same side while walking. Also great for people with scoliosis

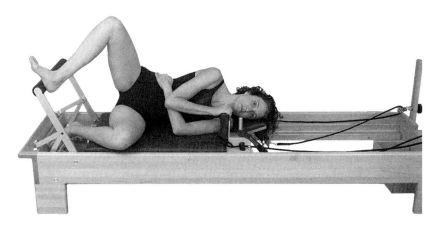

VARIATION: Turn Out 1

Variation: *Turn Out*: Rotate top leg externally (do not allow pelvis to roll back with the leg) and extend the leg, maintaining the turn out

Variation: *Pulses* (not shown): Inhale and push carriage 3" to 5" away from home –or– Pulse carriage in 1–2" range focusing the work on the back of the leg

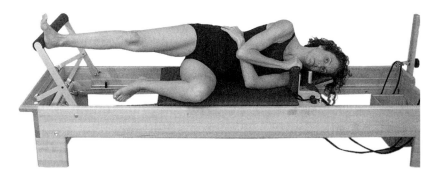

VARIATION: Turn Out 2

MACHINE SET UP
- springs: 2 red
- bar: high or low
- ropes: N/A
- risers: N/A
- headrest: N/A

FUNCTIONS & TARGET MUSCLES
- Strengthens quads and plantar flexors
- Teaches pelvic stabilization
- Stretches hamstrings
- Challenges coordination

ALIGNMENT CUES & OBSTACLES
- Really focus on abdominals stabilizing pelvis as legs move in a large ROM
- Stretch hamstrings before performing this exercise
- Make sure that standing leg stays in parallel, especially when challenged by the big movements of the gesturing leg—keep weight on big toe metatarsal, cueing both the inner thigh and the VMO. Don't turn out!
- **Obstacles:** Tight hamstrings, unstable pelvis

VARIATIONS & PEEL BACKS
- **Variation:** Both legs in turn out, when straightening gesture leg in step 3, you can extend the leg to the side (2nd position in ballet), which really challenges pelvic stability from side to side—keep leg working in 2nd until bending gesture leg into passé at step 8
- **Peel Backs:** *Single Leg Footwork*

IMAGINE...*you are a prima ballerina with the New York City Ballet—feel the precise lines your legs are creating in space.*

ELLIE SAYS...*"It's an 8 count phrase: 'Passé. Développé. Batte...ment. Flex. Point. Passé. Come in.' Cue it like that. Teach those clients some French."*

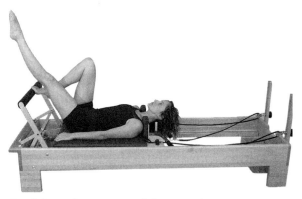

1. Starting Position—*2 to 4 repetitions each leg*
Lying on back with head on the headrest. Place the toes of one leg on footbar and extended other leg over bar.

Inhale to prepare

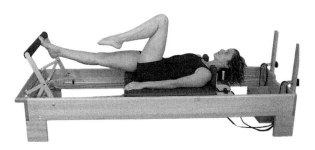

2. Exhale
Pull abs toward spine and push carriage out, straightening working leg while bending the gesture leg, bringing pointed toes to knee. This is passé.

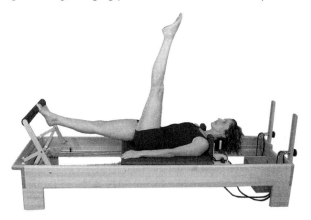

3. Inhale
Straighten gesture leg with toes pointed. Do not tuck pelvis while extending leg. This is développé.

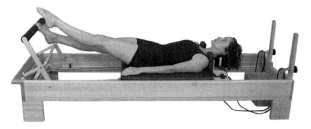

4. Exhale
Lower gesture leg to bar, keeping knees straight. Gently tap footbar with toes.

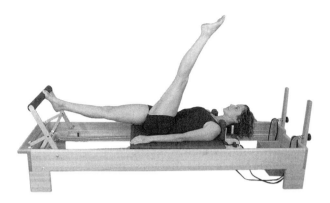

5. Inhale
Quickly raise gesture leg, as if bar is too hot to touch. The lowering and lifting of the leg is the battement.

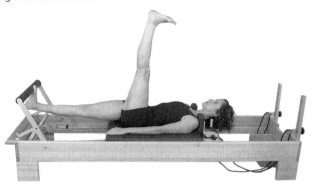

6. Exhale
Flex both feet, standing leg heel goes under bar. Do not let gesture leg lower—in fact, reach its heel higher to increase the hamstring stretch.

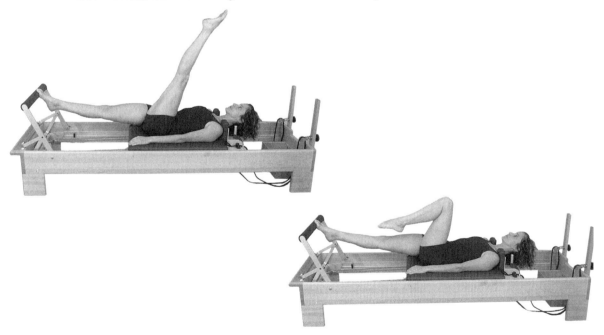

7–9. Inhale/Exhale/Inhale
Point both feet, raising heel of standing leg. Bend knee of gesture leg, bringing toes to the knee of the standing leg—passé. Bend standing leg to bring carriage home while lengthening gesture leg out over the bar, coming back to Starting Position.

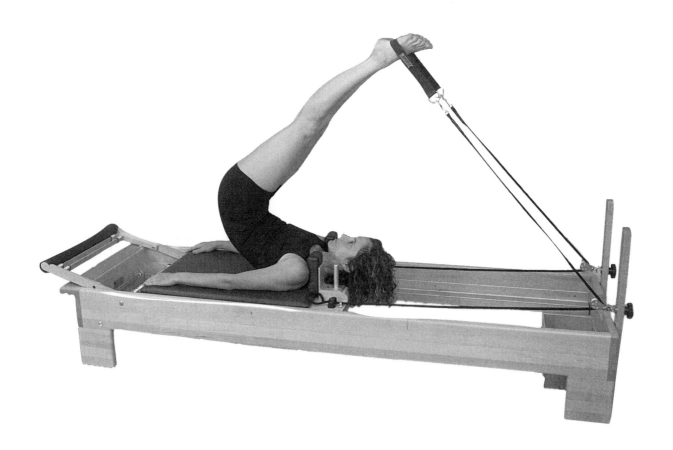

The Supine Series is not a classical series name but simply a way I like to organize the group of exercises that come after *Footwork* and before the Long Box Series. The Supine Series combines beginning arm work with intermediate spine stretches and abdominal exercises. I recommend always including this series in your Reformer workout as it is a great flowing set of exercises that warm up your spine and body, preparing the body for what's to come.

SUPINE: ARMS	**SUPINE: ABDOMINALS**	**SUPINE: SPINE**
Chicken Wings	*The Hundred*	*Frog Extensions*
Lat Pulls	*Coordination*	*Levitation Vérité*
Angels		*Short Spine Stretch*
Triceps		*Overhead/Jackknife*

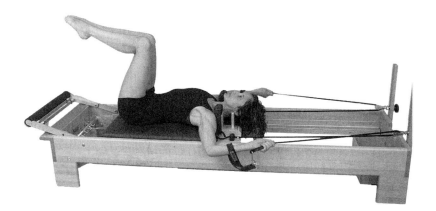

1. Starting Position—*5 repetitions*
Slip hands through the loops and grab onto ropes just above hardware, (you can put the loops around the elbows to reinforce the sensation of pulling from the back). Elbows are bent and even with shoulders. Arms are open and parallel to floor (you will already be in spring resistance with carriage pulled away from home). Legs are in Table Top position, or in towards chest.

Inhale to prepare

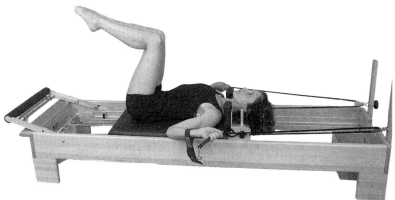

2. Exhale
Pull the elbows down to your imaginary "back pockets," keeping arms parallel to floor and elbows bent.

3. Inhale
Return to Starting Position, controlling carriage and stopping when elbows are even with shoulders.

MACHINE SET UP
- springs: 1 red
- bar: down
- ropes: standard length
- risers: down
- headrest: down

FUNCTIONS & TARGET MUSCLES
- Engages lats while stretching pec major, and chest
- Trains proper shoulder alignment

ALIGNMENT CUES & OBSTACLES
- Keep hands facing away from Reformer and do not let elbows go below carriage
- Do not allow thoracic spine to go into extension (use abdominals to stabilize rib cage) unless...
- If client has really tight pecs, allow some thoracic extension at first
- Keep back of hand magnetized to outer edge of Reformer—wrists stay long
- Keep elbows bent, maintaining "W" position/ shape of arms
- **Contraindications:** Hypermobile shoulders

VARIATIONS & PEEL BACKS
- **Modification:** For injured clients, start on mat or foam roller
- If client is weak in their core, cross ankles and bring femurs closer to chest
- Use Table Top Leg position (shown) to increase abdominal work (but do not allow lumbar spine to hyper-extend)—the further the femurs from the torso, the more abdominal work

IMAGINE...*the rib cage is made of lead to keep ribs from popping...or imagine your arm starts at the scapula and initiate the movement from there.*

ELLIE SAYS...*"Jennifer Stacy, master teacher, developed this exercise many years ago."*

MACHINE SET UP
- springs: 1 red, 1 red and 1 blue, 2 reds
- bar: down
- ropes: standard length
- risers: down
- headrest: down or up

FUNCTIONS & TARGET MUSCLES
- Strengthens lats while stabilizing pelvis and rib cage
- Peel back for *Overhead*
- Teaches Door Frame Arms

ALIGNMENT CUES & OBSTACLES
- Do not allow shoulder to internally rotate so far that the glenohumeral joint loses contact with mat, overworking the pec major
- Feel scapulae sliding down back as arms move
- Keep elbows and wrists straight
- If pecs are overworking, have client widen arms and slightly bend elbows
- If client's kyphotic curve is flat, perform exercise with risers up, cuing them to feel spine between the scapulae making contact with mat

VARIATIONS & PEEL BACKS
- As client gets stronger, increase spring setting
- If client is weak in their core, cross ankles and bring femurs closer to chest
- Use Table Top Leg position (shown) to increase abdominal work (but do not allow lumbar spine to hyper-extend)—the further the femurs from the torso, the more abdominal work

IMAGINE...*your neck is growing away from your body as arms pull down.*

ELLIE SAYS... *"Scapulae are the feet of your arms, and you're standing on your scapulae."*

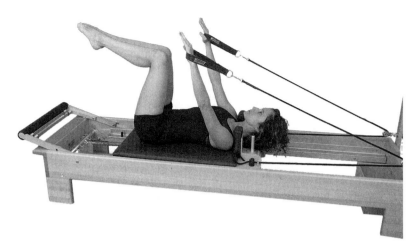

1. Starting Position—*5 repetitions*
Hands in loops or handles with fingers reaching toward the sky. Arms are perpendicular to floor. Back is wide with both scapulae making contact with the mat. Legs are in Table Top position, or in towards chest. Starting Position is already in spring resistance.

Inhale to prepare

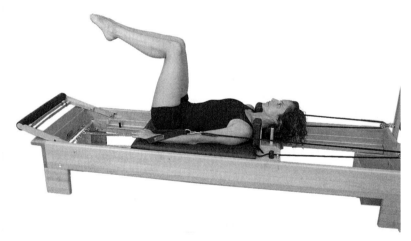

2. Exhale
Engage abdominals while pulling arms down toward carriage until palm makes contact with mat.

3. Inhale
Arms rise back to Starting Position (not home).

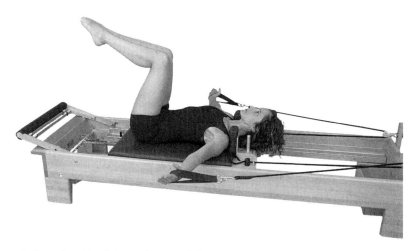

1. Starting Position—*5 repetitions*
Hands in loops with palms toward ceiling. Arms parallel to floor reaching long to either side making a "T" position. Legs are in Table Top position, or in towards chest. Starting Position is already in resistance.

Inhale to prepare

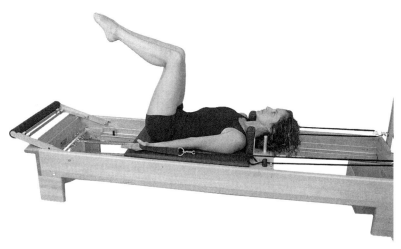

2. Exhale
Pull arms to sides of torso.

3. Inhale
Control carriage to Starting Position (not home).

MACHINE SET UP
- springs: 1 red
- bar: down
- ropes: standard length
- risers: down
- headrest: down or up

FUNCTIONS & TARGET MUSCLES
- Strengthens lats without over-using pec major
- Strengthens teres minor, infraspinatus, and posterior deltoid
- Stabilizes torso with abdominals as arms move
- Begin to feel sense of Serape—serratus anterior/external obliques connection to transversus

ALIGNMENT CUES & OBSTACLES
- Keep clavicles wide as arms move
- Pinkies make contact with torso—keep palms up
- Initiate motion from scapulae, not hands

VARIATIONS & PEEL BACKS
- If client is weak in their core, cross ankles and bring femurs closer to chest
- Use Table Top Leg position (shown) to increase abdominal work (but do not allow lumbar spine to hyper-extend)—the further the femurs from the torso, the more abdominal work
- **Modification:** To find arm motion from back: while arms are close to torso, make 4 small circles initiating from scapula, then reverse direction of circle for 4 more repetitions
- **Variation:** To work abs more, add the beginning of a *Roll Up* as arms pull to sides (really scoop out low abs, flex lumbar spine into mat and go past Pilates Abdominal Position—this is a prep for *The Teaser*)

IMAGINE...*you're making Angels in the snow.*

ELLIE SAYS...*"I can remember making Angels in the snow, way back in Philly...."*

MACHINE SET UP

- springs: 1 or 2 red
- bar: down
- ropes: standard length
- risers: down
- headrest: down or up

FUNCTIONS & TARGET MUSCLES

- Strengthens triceps
- Trains shoulder stabilization

ALIGNMENT CUES & OBSTACLES

- Keep shoulders rotated open and wide on the carriage

VARIATIONS & PEEL BACKS

- If client is weak in their core, cross ankles and bring femurs closer to chest
- Use Table Top Leg position (shown) to increase abdominal work (but do not allow lumbar spine to hyper-extend)—the further the femurs from the torso, the more abdominal work
- **Variation:** Add *Upper Abdominal Curl* as arms pull down to work abdominals, and as a peel back for *The Hundreds,* and *Coordination*

IMAGINE...*that your elbows are glued to the carriage.*

ELLIE SAYS...*"Get that dingle dangle firm."*

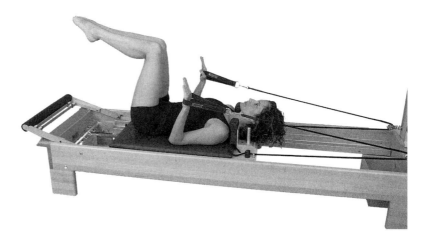

1. Starting Position—*8 to 10 repetitions*
Lie on your back, hands in handles or cotton loops with elbows bent to 90° and fingertips toward ceiling, upper arms glued to sides, legs in Table Top position, or in towards chest.

Inhale to prepare

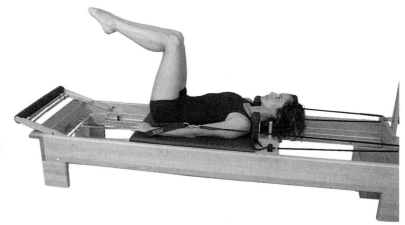

2. Exhale
Scoop abdominals to spine and straighten elbows. Keep knees as straight and legs low as possible while maintaining Abdominal Scoop.

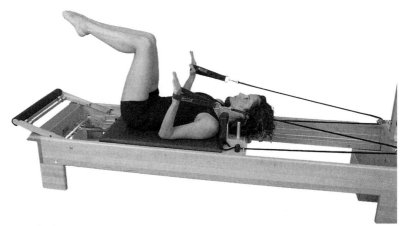

3. Inhale
Bend elbows to 90°, returning to Starting Position.

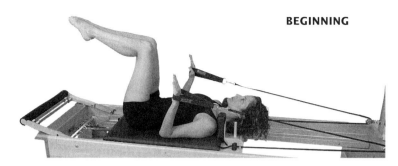

BEGINNING

1. Starting Position—*10 sets of 10 breaths*
Place hands in loops with fingertips toward sky. Elbows are bent to 90°. Legs in Table Top Position. Shoulders about an inch away from shoulder rests.

Inhale to prepare

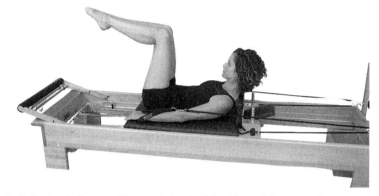

2. Exhale: Roll up to Pilates Abdominal Position while extending arms to sides *(Tricep Press)*.

3–4. Inhale/Exhale
Inhale through nose smoothly for 5 arm pumps. Exhale percussively through the mouth for 5 arm pumps making a "sh–sh" sound. Lumbar spine is deeply imprinted on mat and inner thighs are pulling together.

VARIATIONS:

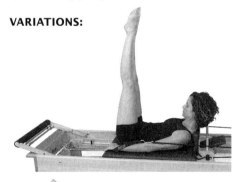

INTERMEDIATE
Legs straight at 90° in Pilates "V"

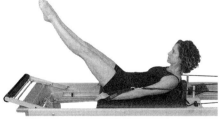

ADVANCED
Legs straight at 45° in Pilates "V"

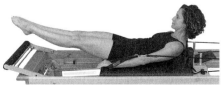

SUPER ADVANCED
Legs straight and low in Pilates "V"
Use your glutes!

MACHINE SET UP
- springs: 1 or 2 red
- bar: down
- ropes: standard length
- risers: down
- headrest: down or up

FUNCTIONS & TARGET MUSCLES
- Warms up the body
- Strengthens abdominal muscles, hip flexors, deep neck flexors, and lats
- Challenges coordination—pump arms in rhythm with breath while maintaining torso stability
- Teaches percussive breathing

ALIGNMENT CUES & OBSTACLES
- On each round of exhales, deepen abdominal engagement and come up higher to maintain Pilates Abdominal Position
- Do not just use rectus abdominis—keep pulling navel to spine to protect the low back
- Maintain Door Frame Arms while pumping, reaching fingers long, pressing into resistance of lats
- Keep upper body stable—do not let upper body rock with arm pumps
- Bring femurs closer to chest to lessen lower abdominal work
- To keep neck relaxed, look to right for one set of breaths and then to left for the next
- **Obstacles:** Weak abs and weak hip flexors, tight upper back

VARIATIONS & PEEL BACKS
- **Intermediate:** Knees straight, legs at 90°, hips in slight external rotation, (this favors the psoas for hip flexion). People with tight hamstrings will have a harder time with this version than the Advanced one
- **Advanced:** Legs straight and externally rotated, dropped to 45°
- **Super Advanced:** once the legs drop below 45°, the glutes are more accessible to help stabilize the pelvis. Make sure to squeeze the glutes when lowering the legs. You may find that this version is actually easier than the Advanced one
- **Variation:** Can perform *Frog Extensions* with legs straightening on each set of exhales to relax hip flexors

IMAGINE...*you are cradling a bowling ball with your spine—so if you're over-using your rectus you're going to pop the ball off your torso. Imagine your sternum is anchored to the mat and you're "hatch-backing" the upper back around this anchor.*

ELLIE SAYS...*"Traditionally The Hundred is a 'warm up' exercise to get the blood circulating."*

FROG EXTENSIONS

MACHINE SET UP
- springs: 2 red, less for smaller clients
- bar: down
- ropes: standard length
- risers: down
- headrest: up or down

FUNCTIONS & TARGET MUSCLES
- Strengthens adductors, quads, hamstrings, and external hip rotators
- Challenges abdominals to maintain Neutral Spine with legs in motion
- Peel back for *Short Spine*

ALIGNMENT CUES & OBSTACLES
- Keep legs at consistent angle—no wavering up and down
- Don't snap knees straight—keep heels together to prevent knee hyperextension
- Don't let hips roll to parallel when knees straighten—use the low glutes
- Keep knees outside of ropes and if ropes are banging into knees, raise legs by flexing more at hips
- Instructors can place hands on client's heels to give resistance and help client feel where their legs are in space

VARIATIONS & PEEL BACKS
- **Variation:** *Parallel Frogs*: Can perform *Frogs* with parallel legs, knees and ankles touching
- **Peel Back:** *Footwork in First Position*

IMAGINE...*you have laser beams shooting out your heels every time the legs straighten.*

ELLIE SAYS...*"This exercise is harder than it looks."*

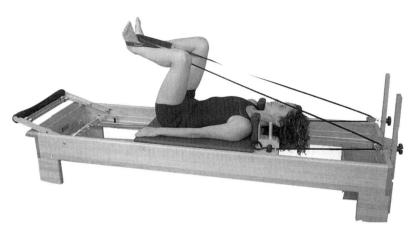

1. Starting Position—*5 repetitions*
Feet in loops. Legs in a *Frog* squat with hips in external rotation, feet flexed with heels together.

Inhale to prepare

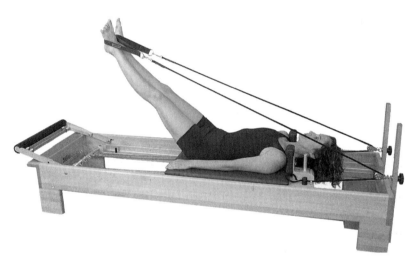

2. Exhale
Feel abdominals pulling toward spine while pressing through the heels as legs straighten on a diagonal (about 45°). Maintain heel connection and Neutral Spine.

3. Inhale
Return to Starting Position, without flexing lumbar spine or losing neutral.

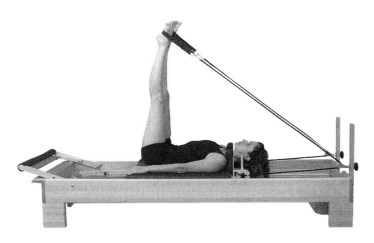

1. Starting Position—*3 to 5 repetitions*
Lying supine with feet in straps, legs at 90° and feet in Pilates "V".

Inhale to prepare

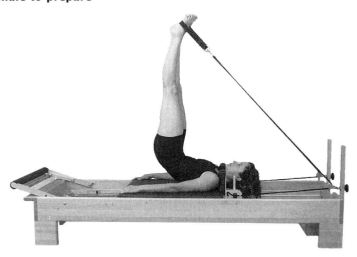

2. Exhale
Pull abdominals to spine to round low back, engage glutes, squeeze inner thighs together and engage rotators (feel the wrap around the upper thigh) to peel pelvis off mat without moving the carriage. Legs stay perpendicular to the floor.

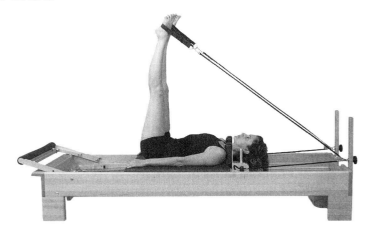

3. Inhale
Control pelvis down to mat.

MACHINE SET UP
- springs: 2 red, less for smaller clients
- bar: down
- ropes: standard
- risers: down
- headrest: down

FUNCTIONS & TARGET MUSCLES
- Teaches the concept of Levitation
- Strengthens glutes, abdominals, and adductors

ALIGNMENT CUES & OBSTACLES
- Keep upper body relaxed and shoulders as open as possible
- Start with small ROM and increase height of pelvis as strength increases
- Do not lower legs in attempt to lift pelvis—legs and pelvis become one unit
- **Obstacles:** tight hamstrings, tight backs
- **Contraindications:** disc dysfunction, osteoporosis, neck injuries

VARIATIONS & PEEL BACKS
- **Variation:** Placing legs in parallel position will use more hamstrings, less glutes and therefore is a little more difficult

IMAGINE...*you're sliding your legs up and down a wall—not just your feet, your entire leg.*

ELLIE SAYS...*"Your client should be able to do this correctly before you teach them Short Spine or Long Spine."*

SHORT SPINE STRETCH

MACHINE SET UP
- springs: 2 red, less for smaller clients
- bar: down
- ropes: standard length
- risers: down
- headrest: down

FUNCTIONS & TARGET MUSCLES
- Stretches spinal muscles
- Teaches sequential movement of spine
- Works abdominals and glutes (in Levitation)

ALIGNMENT CUES & OBSTACLES
- Do not roll up onto cervical spine
- Legs move up and over—not just up, not just over
- Keep neck and shoulders relaxed and do not allow shoulders to roll forward and in
- Do not rely on machine to get pelvis in the air—LEVITATE up
- When rolling down, focus on pelvis moving away from heels with heels remaining stationary
- Make sure carriage is in home position before rolling down
- **Obstacles:** Tight spinal muscles, large lower body
- **Contraindications:** Cervical spine issues, unstable SI joints (it over-stretches back of pelvis), disc dysfunction, osteoporosis

VARIATIONS & PEEL BACKS
- To deepen stretch for clients, place forearm on back of client's thighs and provide gentle pressure as they roll down
- To help clients feel separation of the heels and the pelvis, hold their heels as they roll pelvis down toward carriage
- **Peel Backs:** *Levitation Vérité*, *Frog Extensions*

IMAGINE...*a hot spatula lifts your butt perkily off the carriage.*

ELLIE SAYS...*"Give the clients a stretch. Touch them whenever possible...they'll love you."*

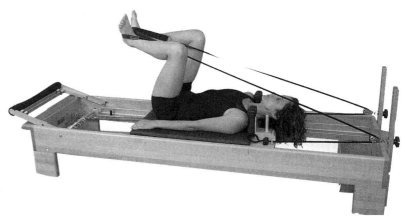

1. Starting Position—*4 repetitions*
Lying on back with loops around arches, legs in *Frog* squat position and arms by sides.

Inhale to prepare

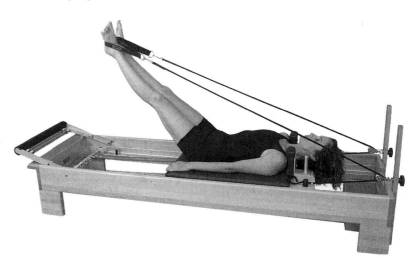

2. Inhale
Straighten legs on diagonal (*Frog Extension*).

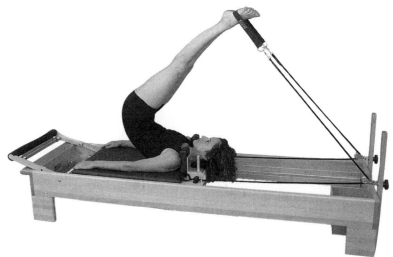

3. Exhale
Flex at hips as legs rise toward body. When they reach 90° hip flexion, use glutes, abdominals and inner thighs to levitate up—pelvis moves up and over head as carriage moves to home. Weight should be between scapulae, not on neck. Anchor the sternum to the mat to avoid pressure on the neck.

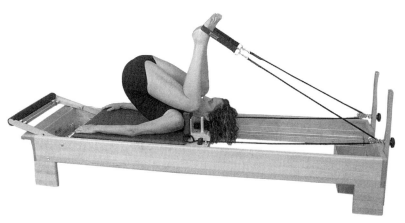

4. Inhale
Keeping carriage still, bend knees down toward shoulder rests—do not splay hips open (body should make a tight ball).

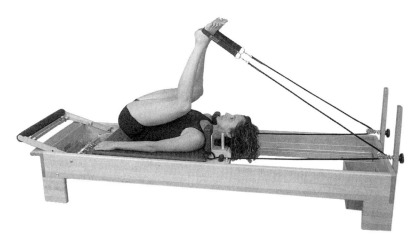

5. Exhale
Pull abdominals toward spine and roll spine down sequentially without moving heels or carriage. Then, still scooping your belly, use hamstrings to pull heels to pelvis and pelvis to the carriage—this will move carriage.

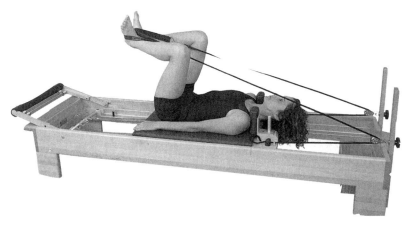

6. Continue to Exhale
Continue pulling pelvis into neutral and legs into *Frog* squat, returning to your Starting Position.

MACHINE SET UP

- springs: 2 red, less for smaller clients
- bar: down
- ropes: standard length
- risers: down
- headrest: down or up

FUNCTIONS & TARGET MUSCLES

- Strengthens abdominal muscles, hip flexors, deep neck flexors, and triceps
- Challenges client coordination—legs move independently of arms

ALIGNMENT CUES & OBSTACLES

- Perform this exercise with finesse and control with accent on the "in" motion as legs open and close
- Maintain Pilates Abdominal Positioning— no decrease in spinal flexion, no dropping or juicing the imaginary fruit between chin and chest

VARIATIONS & PEEL BACKS

- **Variation:** When knees are straight add *Running* or *Scissor* legs from Leg Spring series—legs go only as low as Abdominal Scoop can be maintained and lumbar spine stays slightly flexed
- **Peel Backs:** *Tricep Presses*, then add *Tricep Presses* with simultaneous upper abdominal curl
- Increase springs to work triceps more
- It is easier on the neck to keep the head up rather than lifting and lowering the head with each repetition—if client has neck issues have them try the exercise keeping head down and just moving arms and legs, then add 1 or 2 repetitions with head raising into Pilates Abdominal Position

IMAGINE...*you can move your arms separately from your legs!*

ELLIE SAYS...*"Cue it like this: Extend... Open...Close...Knees...Arms."*

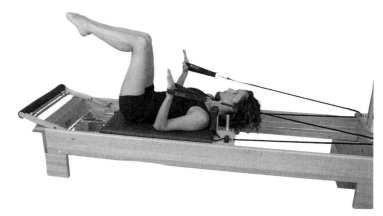

1. Starting Position—*5 or 6 repetitions*
Hands in loops with elbows bent to 90° and fingertips toward ceiling, upper arms glued to sides, legs in Table Top position.

Inhale to prepare

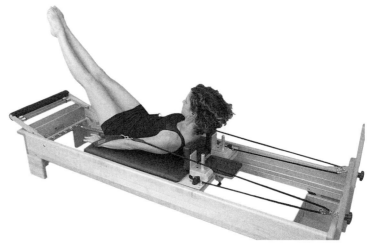

2. Percussive Exhale
Scoop abdominals to spine while simultaneously straightening elbows and knees, raise head and upper back into Pilates Abdominal Position. Palms touch the mat and legs go out on a diagonal as low as Abdominal Scoop can be maintained and lumbar spine stays in contact with mat.

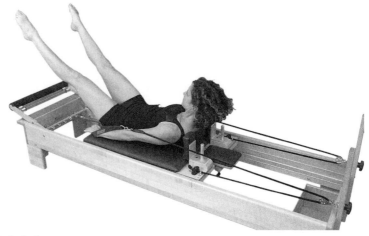

3. Inhale
Open legs to width of the carriage.

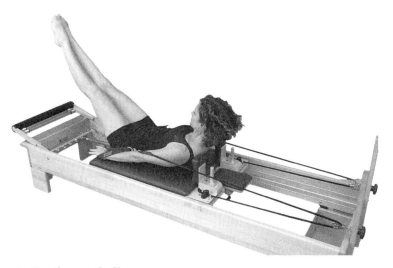

4. Continue Inhaling
Close legs quickly.

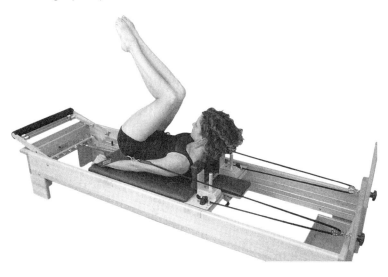

5. Exhale
Bend knees toward chest and do small *Hip Up*.

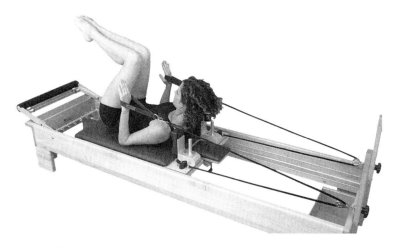

6. Inhale
Bend elbows to 90°—elbows stay on mat—maintaining Pilates Abdominal Position.

MACHINE SET UP
- springs: 2 red, less for smaller clients
- bar: down
- ropes: standard length
- risers: down
- headrest: down

FUNCTIONS & TARGET MUSCLES
- Strengthens abdominals, lats, and triceps
- Trains Levitation and control
- Stretches the spine

ALIGNMENT CUES & OBSTACLES
- Do not roll up onto cervical spine, instead roll onto your Thoracic Shelf, balancing between your shoulder blades
- Legs move up and over—not just up, not just over
- Keep neck and shoulders relaxed—do not allow shoulders to roll forward and in
- When rolling down focus on pelvis moving away from heels with heels remaining stationary
- Make sure carriage is in home position before rolling down
- **Obstacles:** Tight spinal muscles, tight hamstrings, large lower body, weak abdominals
- **Contraindications:** disc dysfunction, osteoporosis and/or neck injuries

VARIATIONS & PEEL BACKS
- **Peel Backs:** *Lat Pulls, Roll Over* on the Mat

IMAGINE...*your legs are as light as popsicle sticks as you levitate them up and over your head.*

ELLIE SAYS...*"Now that's Levitation."*

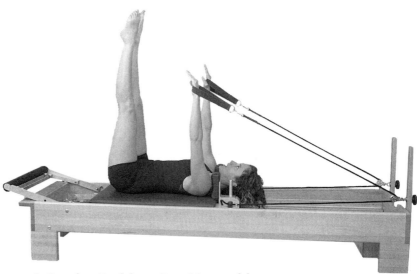

1. Starting Position—*8 to 10 repetitions*
Lie on your back, hands in loops with arms and legs reaching up to the sky, legs in Pilates First Position.

Inhale to prepare

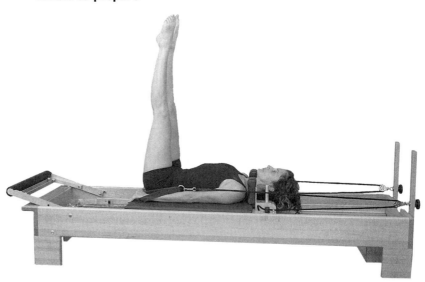

2. Exhale
Do a *Lat Pull*, so that your Door Frame Arms press down onto the carriage.

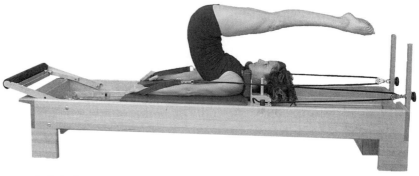

3. Inhale
Lift your hips up and over your head, ending with legs parallel to the floor (no lower).

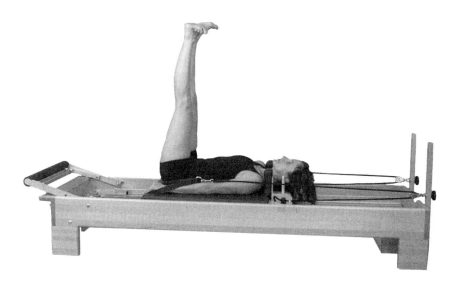

4. Exhale
Flex your feet and reach long through your heels to roll down one vertebra at a time, until your legs reach back up to the sky.

5. Inhale
Allow your arms to retrograde, reaching fingertips back up to the sky to return to Starting Position.

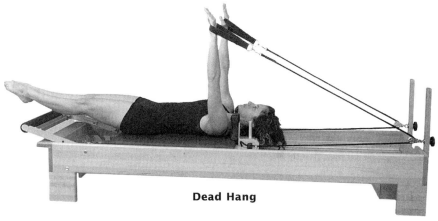

Dead Hang

VARIATION: Dead Hang
Add a *Dead Hang* to the intermediate *Overhead* by lowering your legs (only as far as you can maintain a flat lower back on the mat) while your arms are coming up to the sky. Then lift your legs up to the sky as your arms do a *Lat Pull* down onto the carriage. "Legs lower as arms lift, then legs lift as arms lower."

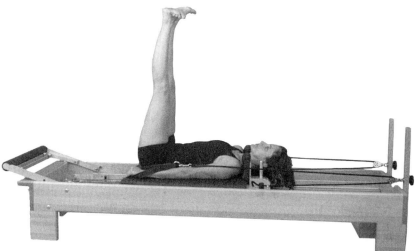

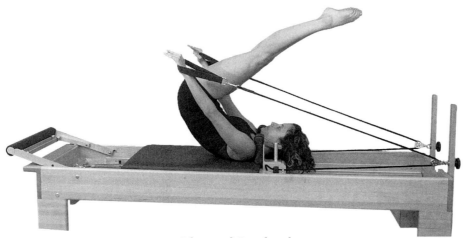

Advanced Overhead

Simultaneously initiate the *Lat Pull* and the Levitation so that the arms reach the carriage at the same time as the legs finish their overhead ascent. Note: Start levitating the hips first on the way up, and then activate the arms a nano second later. On the descent, start lifting the arms first by reaching into the lats. Do this by lengthening the fingers long away from you, and then follow with the hips rolling down. You still want to have the arms and the legs arrive at the end of each movement at the same time. Add the *Dead Hang* to this version, keeping your arms in a space-hold, reaching up to the sky, as you lower your legs to the dead hang and back up to 90° angle to start again.

Lighten the resistance for more Levitation challenge!

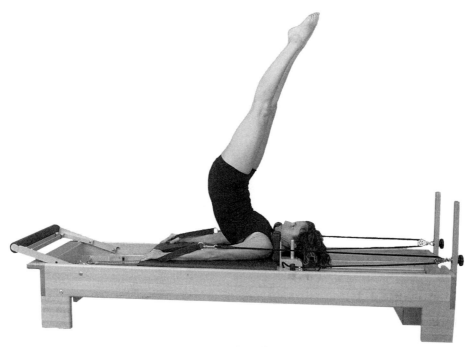

Jackknife

Once you are in your *Overhead* position, with Door Frame Arms pressing into the carriage, simply levitate your hips to the sky, and then fold back in half and continue the exercise. This is the *Jackknife* movement. Do not roll onto your neck, but try to stay on your Thoracic Shelf instead.

Contraindications: disc dysfunction, osteoporosis and/or neck injuries

rowing series

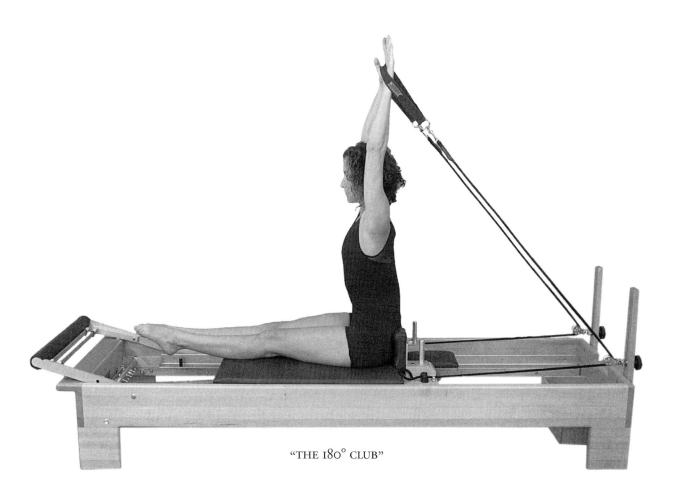

"THE 180° CLUB"

The main purpose of the Rowing Series is to strengthen the shoulder girdle, train proper alignment of the shoulder, and increase Range of Motion. The Advanced Rowing Combos are complicated in their choreography and require lots of practice to keep the all the movements flowing and connected.

These are the first seated exercises in the Reformer Series, so check for proper seated posture. If Pilates does anything for people, it teaches them how to sit and stand properly, strengthening their postural muscles. When seated, make sure that clients are perfectly stacked with head atop shoulders, shoulders atop hips. The lower back should have it's natural lumbar curve; the pelvis should be neutral. Give your clients a pillow or wedge to sit on if they have difficulty achieving this perfection. For clients with limited flexibility, put them up on the long box.

BEGINNING	**INTERMEDIATE**	**ADVANCED COMBOS**
Hug a Tree	*Salute*	*Front Rowing*
Modified Front Rowing		*Back Rowing: Round Back*
		Back Rowing: Flat Back Hinge

MACHINE SET UP

- springs: 1 blue or 1 red
- bar: down
- ropes: standard length
- risers: down
- headrest: N/A

FUNCTIONS & TARGET MUSCLES

- Strengthens deltoids and pec major
- Works abdominals and postural muscles
- Teaches scapular stabilization with humeral motion (mid traps, serratus anterior, rhomboids)

ALIGNMENT CUES & OBSTACLES

- Keep skull aligned over pelvis in excellent sitting posture while moving arms
- Sit right on sit bones—no slouching behind them or arching in front of them
- Feel chest and back staying wide and stable as arms move
- Reach through pinky finger to encourage the serratus anterior to work
- As arms return to Starting Position do not let elbows move behind torso—this will pinch shoulder blades and force pecs to initiate the next "hug"
- Pull the head of the humerus back in the shoulder socket to cue the back muscles and get out of the pecs
- Think: ballet arms

VARIATIONS & PEEL BACKS

- To increase difficulty, sit with legs straight in front of you
- To work arm strength use red spring
- **Modification:** If client is unable to sit up straight in cross-legged position place them on a moon box, mat, or pillow, or wedge
- **Modification:** For clients who cannot sit cross legged at all, do the whole series on a long box, legs straddling the box, and make sure to rise the ropes up on the risers to accommodate for this change in height
- **Variation**: *Butterfly:* Try this same exercise but with the arms straight

IMAGINE...*you're Shiva and you have 2 extra sets of arms, with one set attached to your scapulae and the other set attached to your rib cage. Hug the tree with all 6 of your arms.*

ELLIE SAYS...*"Romana used to call this Hug Pavarotti."*

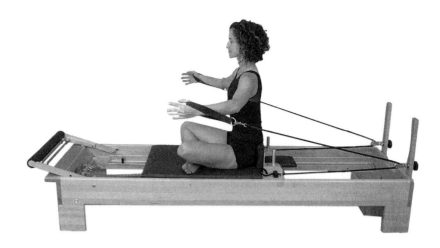

1. Starting Position—*6 repetitions*

Sit cross-legged on carriage facing front of Reformer with back against shoulder rests. Hands in loops with arms to sides with hands and elbows slightly lower than shoulders. Elbows are slightly rounded. Arms are slightly in front of torso. You should be able to see your elbows with your peripheral vision. These are "ballet arms."

Inhale and lengthen spine

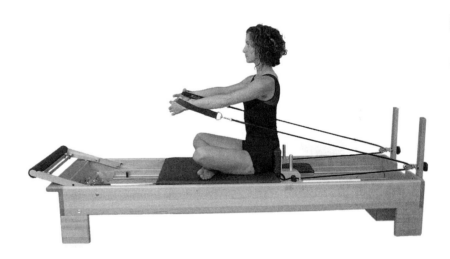

2. Exhale

Keeping back wide and spine long, pull hands toward one another as if you were hugging a tree. Keep elbows rounded.

3. Inhale

Open arms to Starting Position, growing ever taller in spine.

After 3 repetitions **reverse the breathing** so the arms pull together. Inhale for 3 more repetitions. Breathe into the serratus anterior as you initiate the hug.

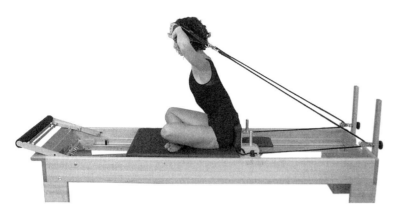

1. Starting Position—*6 repetitions (3 of each variation)*
Transition from *Hug a Tree, Salute* forehead with elbows bent, and index fingers touching eyebrows with palms facing out. Torso is pitched forward about 20° from upright.

Inhale to prepare

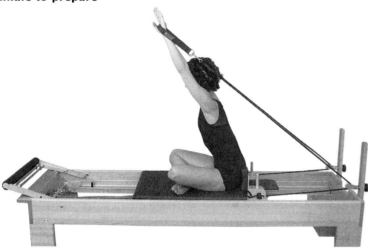

2–3. Exhale/Inhale
Straighten elbows while stabilizing scapulae so they don't elevate. Arms straighten to Door Frame position on the line of the body. Hands are even with or wider than shoulders. Inhale. Elbows bend and fingers return to eyebrows. Repeat 3 times.

Shave the Head

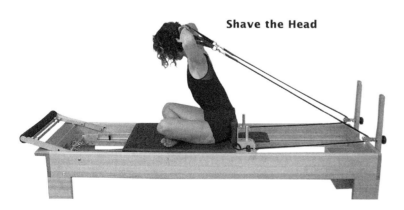

4–5. Exhale/Inhale
On 4th rep, drop head forward bringing hands behind head and *Salute* the Pilates goddess from this position (like you're shaving off the back of your head). Inhale. Return to Starting Position with control. Repeat 3 times.

MACHINE SET UP
- springs: 1 blue or 1 red
- bar: down
- ropes: standard length
- risers: down
- headrest: N/A

FUNCTIONS & TARGET MUSCLES
- Strengthens triceps, deltoids, and back extensors
- Teaches shoulder girdle stability

ALIGNMENT CUES & OBSTACLES
- Keep shoulders wide and scapulae sliding down back—do not overuse upper traps!
- If it is difficult to keep shoulders down, allow arms to widen as they extend—saluting more toward the side than the front
- **Obstacles:** Tight upper traps and lats
- **Contraindication:** Carpal Tunnel Syndrome, and upper quarter Repetitive Stress Injury issues (it is very difficult not to overuse upper traps and levator scapula)

VARIATIONS & PEEL BACKS
- **Modification:** Tight hips and/or a tight low back make it difficult to hinge forward—in this case have client sit on mat, pillow, or moon box
- **Modification:** For clients who cannot sit cross-legged at all, do the whole series on a long box, legs straddling the box, and make sure to rise the ropes up on the risers to accommodate for this change in height
- **Peel Back:** *Double Lat Pulls* on the Cadillac (both versions)
- To increase difficulty, sit with legs straight in front of you
- To work arm strength use red spring

IMAGINE... *you are Saluting the Pilates goddess.*

SUSI SAYS... *"I rarely see this exercise done correctly. So don't teach it to your clients until they can stabilize their shoulders while raising their arms above their heads seated upright. That pitch forward truly increases the difficulty of this exercise."*

MODIFIED FRONT ROWING

MACHINE SET UP
- springs: 1 blue or 1 red
- bar: down
- ropes: standard length
- risers: down
- headrest: N/A

FUNCTIONS & TARGET MUSCLES
- Strengthens deltoids
- Strengthens abdominals and postural muscles
- Teaches scapular stabilization and works mid traps, serratus anterior, rhomboids
- Peel back for *Front Rowing Combo*

ALIGNMENT CUES & OBSTACLES
- With every inhale, lengthen spine and maintain that length with every exhale—using abdominals, of course
- Feel scapulae sliding down back as arms raise
- Feel pinkies cut through space as you lower arms to sides—staying in the "side seam" of your torso, not forward!
- Feel lats stretch as arms rise above head
- Widen arms if necessary to keep shoulders down while raising arms above head
- Do not sacrifice rib cage stability to align arms with spine—don't let ribs poke out
- **Obstacles:** Tight lats and upper traps

VARIATIONS & PEEL BACKS
- **Modification:** If client is unable to sit up straight in crossed-legged position, place them on a moon box, mat, or pillow
- **Modification:** For clients who cannot sit cross-legged at all, do the whole series on a long box, legs straddling the box, and make sure to rise the ropes up on the risers to accommodate for this change in height
- To increase difficulty, sit with legs straight in front of you
- To work arm strength use red spring

IMAGINE...*your head is poking through the clouds every time you lower your arms.*

ELLIE SAYS...*"In order to do Pilates with perfect form, it is essential to belong to the 180° Club (shoulders able to flex so that they are in line with the torso). Also the 90° Club (hips are able to flex to 90° when knees are straight)."*

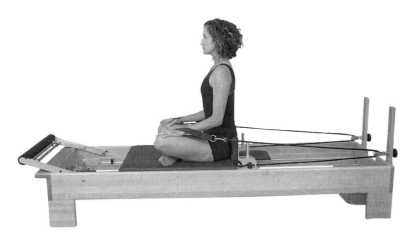

1. Starting Position—*4 repetitions*
Sit cross-legged on carriage facing front of Reformer with back against shoulder rests. Hands are placed in loops resting on knees. Transition from *Salute* by reaching arms straight up and then open to the sides. Sneak your hands onto your knees (see steps 4–7 of this exercise).

Inhale to lengthen spine

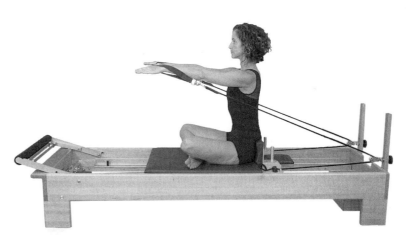

2. Exhale
Pull abdominals toward spine, stabilize scapulae and straighten arms while raising them to 90° at shoulder height, shaving off the tops of the knees.

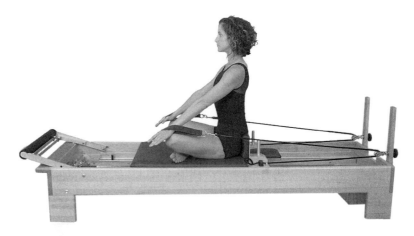

3. Inhale
Lengthen spine while lowering arms, bringing hands back to knees.

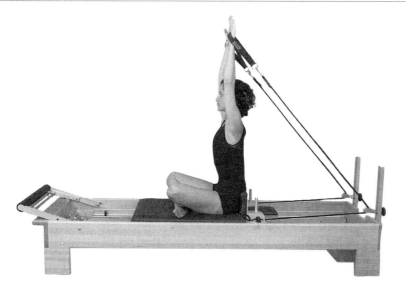

4. Exhale
Pull abdominals toward spine, stabilize scapulae and straighten elbows while raising arms above head (widen arms if necessary to keep shoulders away from ears)—making one long line from tailbone to top of head (180° Club).

5. Inhale
Sit up tall.

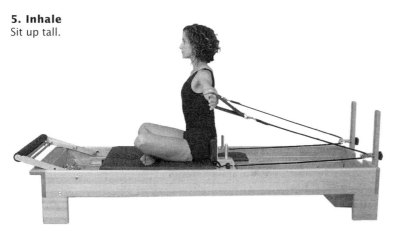

6. Exhale
Spine grows taller as arms open to sides, with your pinkies, bringing arms all the way down to the hips, cutting through your imaginary side seam.

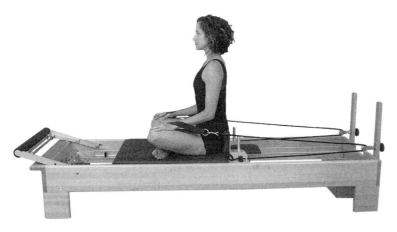

7. Inhale
Sneak hands back to top of knees to start again.

FRONT ROWING

MACHINE SET UP
- springs: 1 blue or 1 red
- bar: down
- ropes: standard length
- risers: down
- headrest: N/A

FUNCTIONS & TARGET MUSCLES
- Strengthens shoulder stabilizers
- Stretches lats, spinal erectors, and hamstrings
- Challenges coordination and memory

ALIGNMENT CUES & OBSTACLES
- As always, keep upper traps as relaxed as possible and keep scapulae stable on a wide back, not elevated toward ears
- Feel energy shooting out of heels when feet are flexed and out of toes when feet are pointed
- Do not collapse to bend forward—lengthen spine as if you were curving over a beach ball
- Try to keep elbows straight throughout exercise
- **Obstacles:** Tight hamstrings, tight lats, weak psoas
- **Contraindications:** disc dysfunction, osteoporosis

VARIATIONS & PEEL BACKS
- **Peel Backs:** *Modified Front Rowing, Salute*

IMAGINE...on the last movement (step 6), you are cutting through the air with your pinkies.

ELLIE SAYS..."Since the Advanced Rowing combos contain intricate movements and complex choreography, they are some of the hardest Pilates exercises to memorize. So practice them regularly until they are emblazoned on your cortex."

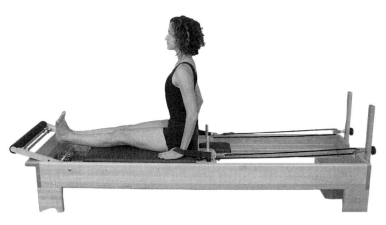

1. Starting Position—*3 to 4 repetitions*
Sit upright with back against the shoulder rests, facing front of Reformer. Legs are extended in front of body with ankles, knees, and inner thighs touching. Hands are in loops with arms by sides and palms resting on carriage.

Inhale, lengthen spine to prepare

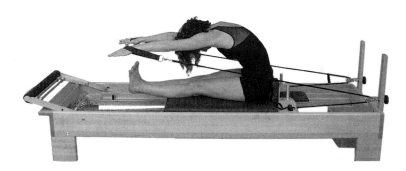

2. Exhale
Flex feet, pull abdominals to spine and bend forward, rounding spine, bringing nose toward knees. Slide hands along carriage reaching arms toward toes.

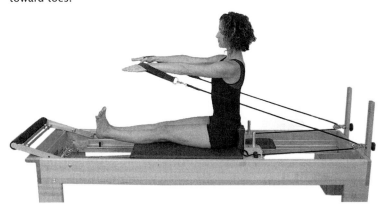

3. Inhale
Stack spine sequentially from tail to head bringing arms up with torso, fingers reach forward with straight elbows. Hands are in line with shoulders and palms remain toward floor. Keep back wide and pecs relaxed. "Ka-chunk" the humerus into the back.

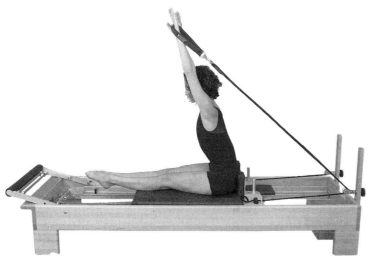

4. Exhale

Point feet and pitch forward hinging at hips, reaching from base of spine, raising arms up as torso stretches diagonally forward, creating one line from tailbone to fingertips. Torso moves forward and arms reach up, meeting in the middle creating the *Salute* position. Keep scapulae stable. Keep low back neutral.

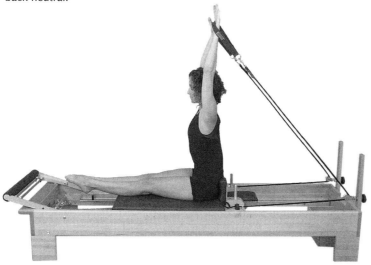

5. Inhale

Bring upper body upright in one piece. Fingers reach toward ceiling with energy shooting out of top of head, shoulders remain connected to back. (180° Club plus 90° Club!)

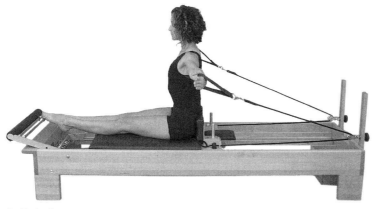

6. Exhale

Leading with pinky fingers, open arms wide to the sides. Spine grows taller as pinkies cut through air and return to sides with hands resting on the carriage.

BACK ROWING: ROUND BACK

MACHINE SET UP
- springs: 1 blue or 1 red
- bar: down
- ropes: standard length
- risers: down
- headrest: down

FUNCTIONS & TARGET MUSCLES
- Strengthens shoulder stabilizers
- Stretches spinal erectors and works abdominals
- Stretches shoulders and arms
- Challenges coordination and memory

ALIGNMENT CUES & OBSTACLES
- Really use abdominals to resist movement of carriage when bending forward or rolling up to enhance spine stretch
- In the starting arm position elbows are bent just enough to feel upper back widen without over engaging pecs
- **Contraindications:** disc dysfunction, osteoporosis

VARIATIONS & PEEL BACKS
- If calves feel cramped by shoulder rests, cross the ankles
- **Peel Back:** *Round Back Roll Down*

IMAGINE...*you are a bird of prey about to pounce as your arms fly around to the front.*

SUSI SAYS...*"This version of rowing always reminds of the dying swan from the Swan Lake. So execute Round Back Rowing with finesse and a sense of drama."*

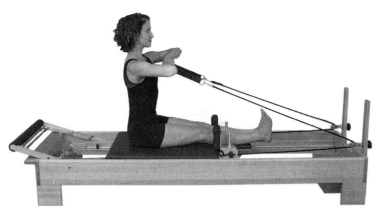

1. Starting Position—*3 repetitions*
Sit upright facing back of Reformer, legs extended straight in front with calves resting on headrest. Hands hold the loops making soft fists with elbows bending into a diamond shape. Feet are flexed.

Inhale and engage low glutes, lengthening torso away from pelvis

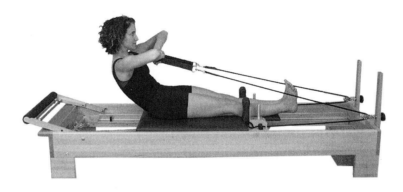

2. Exhale
Pull abdominals to spine, reach through heels and round lumbar spine, pulling torso behind sit bones, rolling about halfway way down.

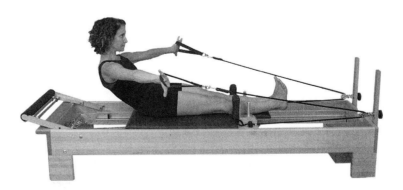

3. Inhale
Maintain C-Curve of spine, and without moving the carriage, open arms to sides by hinging from elbows. Keep scapulae engaged down back.

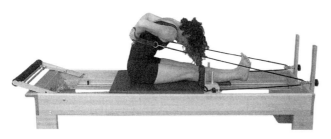

4. Exhale
Increase abdominal engagement, hollowing out the front of the body to bring upper body through arms as they circle around behind the back in a kind of grandiose breaststroke action—the body then begins to fold in half. Reaching arms behind torso, slowly round spine forward, bringing the nose toward the knees and clasping hands behind back, interlacing fingers, palms facing the back. Then bend elbows, bringing hands toward body.

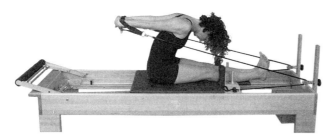

5. Inhale
Straighten arms, rotating the shoulders open, keeping everything else perfectly still.

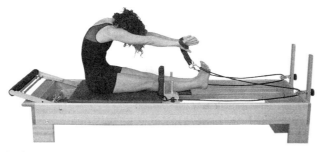

6. Exhale
Release hands without "popping." Circle arms forward, pulling abdominals deeply to spine to round forward. Arms continue circling until they are parallel and the back of hands face one another. This is your "bird of prey" moment—really accentuate the thoracic C-Curve.

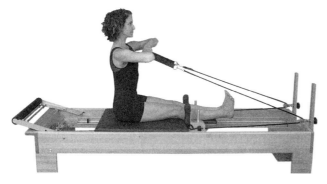

7. Inhale
Stack up from base of spine coming into seated upright position, bending elbows bringing back of hands together, moving hands toward sternum to create a diamond shape. Squeeze low glutes to lift up tall in preparation for repeating the exercise.

BACK ROWING: FLAT BACK HINGE

MACHINE SET UP
- springs: 1 blue or 1 red
- bar: down
- ropes: standard length
- risers: down
- headrest: down

FUNCTIONS & TARGET MUSCLES
- Strengthens shoulder stabilizers and spinal erectors
- Works abdominals and stretches hamstrings
- Challenges memory, coordination, and control

ALIGNMENT CUES & OBSTACLES
- Really use abdominals to lengthen and stabilize spine
- Perform exercise with as much finesse and control as you can muster
- Lift slightly through sternum while hinging back and feel the chest open to the sky
- **Obstacles:** Tight hamstrings, weak psoas

VARIATIONS & PEEL BACKS
- If calves feel cramped by shoulder rests, cross the ankles
- **Peel Backs:** *Flat Back Roll Down, Chest Expansion*

IMAGINE...that you're throwing rice toward the ceiling as you straighten arms while hinging forward.

ELLIE SAYS...*"This is the only supraspinatus exercise in the Pilates repertoire (step 7)."*

SUSI SAYS...*"This version of Rowing has an early modern dance feel, reminiscent of Doris Humphrey's movement theory of the arc between two deaths."*

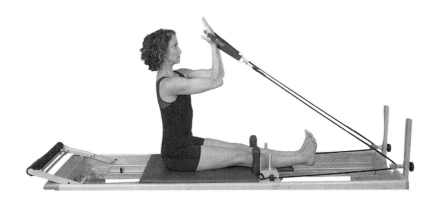

1. Starting Position—*3 repetitions*
Seated upright facing back of Reformer, knees are straight with legs extended through headrest. Arms are in front of the body with hands through loops. The elbows are bent to 90° and even with the shoulders to form "Pilates elbows." Palms face the body with fingers long. Feet are flexed. Pull the head of the humerus back in the shoulder socket.

Inhale and engage low glutes lengthening torso away from pelvis

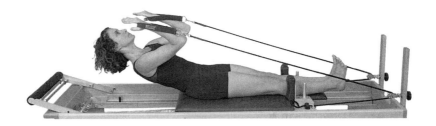

2–3. Exhale/Inhale
Pull abdominals to spine and hinge backwards, lifting chest slightly while performing a bicep curl, keeping elbows high. Go back as far as you feel safe—and watch that you don't go so far that you fall into the well. Inhale, keeping sternum lifted.

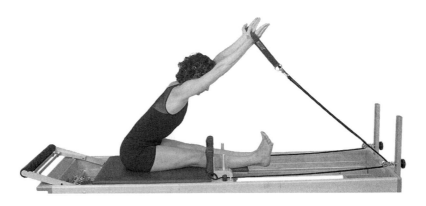

4. Exhale
Straighten elbows, reaching arms toward ceiling as you hinge forward. Folding at the hip, reach arms away from shoulders to increase length in the spine. Keep spine long and straight for as long as possible.

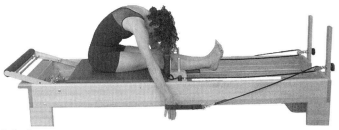

5. Inhale

Allow spine to round when necessary, bringing nose to knees and lowering arms outside of carriage. Arms will finish outside the wood of the Reformer.

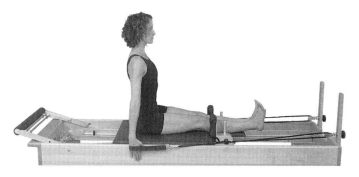

6–7. Exhale/Inhale

Stack up spine from bottom to top while simultaneously performing *Chest Expansion,* ending seated upright, bringing arms even with torso and palms facing wood. Feel collarbones widen as shoulders open and spine unfurls to lengthened position. Inhale and hold this *Chest Expansion* moment.

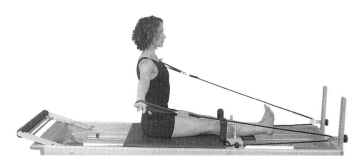

8. Exhale

Stabilize scapulae and internally rotate humerus. Keeping the carriage still, raise arms out to the sides, leading with pinkies until arms are just below shoulder height. Keep shoulders away from ears. Arms should be slightly in front of the body.

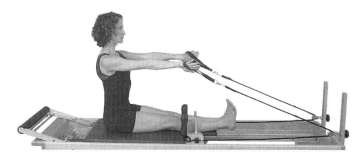

9–10. Inhale/Exhale

Keeping arms parallel to the floor, pull arms forward, leading with the backs of the hands. Exhale and flip hands and bend elbows bringing arms back into Starting Position.

long box series

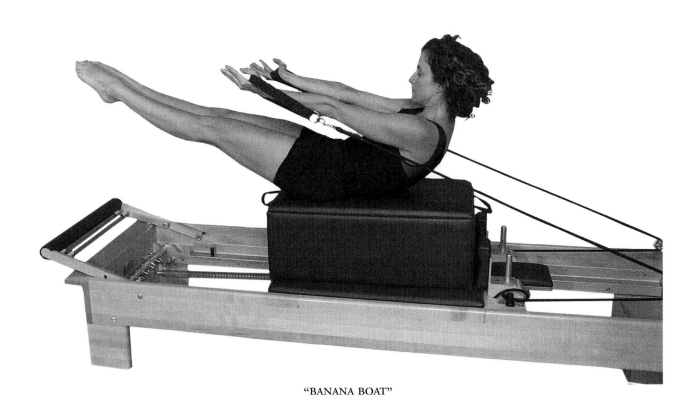

"BANANA BOAT"

The Long Box Series combines shoulder and back strengthening exercises with some of the most advanced abdominal exercises in the repertoire. The seated exercises focus on shoulder stabilization. More advanced versions of these exercises are done kneeling. The prone exercises focus on shoulder stabilization and upper back extension—great for people with rounded shoulders and hunchback posture. *Charlie Chaplin, Swimming Legs,* and *Hamstrings* are some of the best exercises for the butt and back of legs. The supine exercises are some of the most challenging abdominal exercises known to mankind: the *Backstroke,* and of course, the infamous *Teaser!*

SEATED LONG BOX SERIES	**PRONE LONG BOX SERIES**	**SUPINE LONG BOX SERIES**
Chest Expansion	*Pulling Ropes*	*Backstroke*
La Croix	*The "T"*	*Balance Point*
Rotator	*Triceps*	*Teaser*
The Queen	*Hamstrings*	
	Charlie Chaplin	
	Swimming	
	Rocking Swan	
	Grasshopper	

For extra added fun, try the *Fives* on the Long Box!

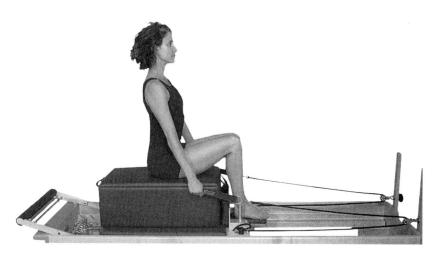

1. Starting Position—*4 to 8 repetitions*
Sit up straight and tall with hands holding loops, pinkies facing back, elbows straight and shoulders relaxed.

Inhale to prepare

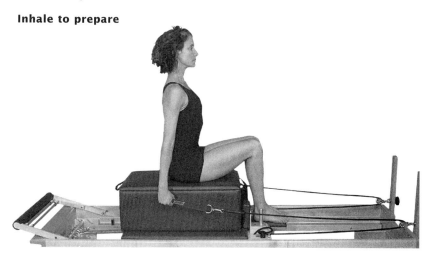

2. Exhale
Stabilize rib cage with the abdominals and pull arms back, opening the chest, pulling the head of the humerus back in the socket, until arms are even with or just slightly behind torso, shoulder blades sliding down the back.

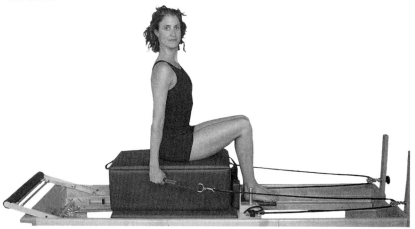

3–4. Inhale/Exhale/Inhale
Rotate head side to side, then back to front for a gentle stretch of the neck. Keep torso stable while looking to each side—don't rotate from rib cage or shoulders. Control arms back to Starting Position, maintaining torso stability.

MACHINE SET UP
- springs: 1 blue or 1 red
- bar: N/A
- ropes: standard length
- risers: down
- headrest: down, with sticky pad

FUNCTIONS & TARGET MUSCLES
- Strengthens the lats, triceps, and posterior deltoids
- Works scapula stabilizers and abdominals
- Peel back for *Kneeling Chest Expansion* and *Flat Back Rowing*

ALIGNMENT CUES & OBSTACLES
- Maintain length of spine and torso stability while arms pull back
- Keep neck relaxed and shoulders down—feel collar bones widen to pull arms to sides
- Place a pole against client's spine for postural feedback (forward head, slouching, and/or torso instability)
- Roll shoulder open from the head of the humerus
- Don't let rib cage pop-out as shoulders open—this is the "fight of the pecs"

VARIATIONS & PEEL BACKS
- **Variation:** *Kneeling* (Intermediate) (see page 128)

IMAGINE…*initiating the arm pull from the abdominals to keep rib cage over pelvis. Imagine you're in a boat trying to skim the water with your fingers tips.*

ELLIE SAYS…*"This is the perfect alignment exercise."*

MACHINE SET UP
- springs: 1 blue or 1 red
- bar: N/A
- ropes: standard length
- risers: down
- headrest: down, with sticky pad

FUNCTIONS & TARGET MUSCLES
- Strengthens rhomboids and mid-traps
- Peel back for *Roll Downs—Rhomboids Variation*
- Stabilizes shoulders

ALIGNMENT CUES & OBSTACLES
- Initiate movement by pulling scapulae together, not by pulling elbows back
- Keep motion small and concentrated between shoulder blades
- Do not try to keep shoulders down, since rhomboids elevate shoulders
- Maintain shape of arms as scapulae pull together
- Great exercise for kyphotic clients and/or breast-feeding mothers

VARIATIONS & PEEL BACKS
- **Modification:** If rhomboids are extremely weak, or client is recovering from shoulder injury, use the yellow spring and focus on the scapulae gliding together and apart
- **Variation:** *Kneeling* (Intermediate) (see page 129)

IMAGINE...*there is a rubber band stretched taut between your shoulder blades. When the rubber band is released into a slackened position, it moves the blades closer together.*

SUSI SAYS...*"On a rehab note—this is the perfect exercise for clients with Thoracic Outlet Syndrome."*

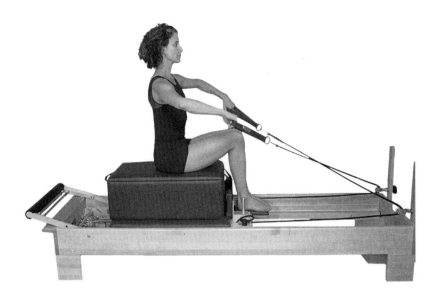

1. Starting Position—*4 to 8 repetitions*
Sitting up straight and tall with ropes crossed, hands holding loops with elbows bent and opened to the sides, making a diamond shape with arms. Hands are below sternum.

Inhale and lengthen spine

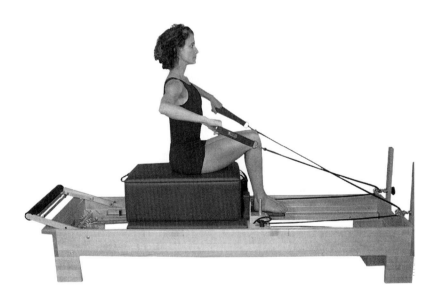

2–3. Exhale/Inhale
Pull abdominals to spine, stabilizing the rib cage, and gently squeeze scapulae together, maintaining diamond shape of arms. Inhale as you return to Starting Position. Relax rhomboids, allowing scapulae to glide apart.

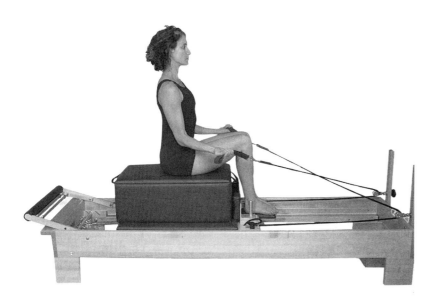

1. Starting Position—*4 to 8 repetitions*
Sit up straight and tall with ropes crossed, loops held with palms up and loop ends next to thumbs—the "hitch-hiker hold." Elbows bent to 90° and glued to sides.

Inhale and lengthen spine

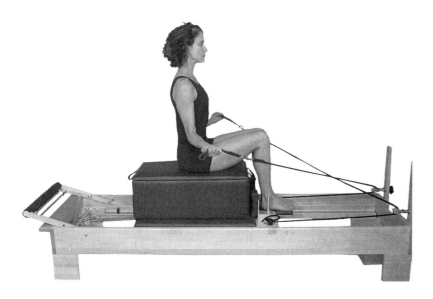

2–3. Exhale/Inhale
Stabilize rib cage by pulling abdominals toward spine. Roll humerus back, allowing forearms to rotate to sides, keeping forearms parallel to floor. Elbows do not move away from sides. Inhale. Control arms back slowly to Starting Position.

MACHINE SET UP
- springs: 1 yellow, 1 blue or 1 red
- bar: N/A
- ropes: standard length
- risers: down
- headrest: down, with sticky pad

FUNCTIONS & TARGET MUSCLES
- Strengthens infraspinatus and teres minor—external rotators of the shoulder joint
- Works postural muscles and abdominals
- Opens chest and shoulders
- Stabilizes shoulder joint

ALIGNMENT CUES & OBSTACLES
- Initiate the movement from the back of the shoulder—do not pull with hands
- Feel humerus rolling backward to make the hands move away from each other
- Do not allow elbows to pull away from torso (that recruits the deltoid)
- Do not allow forearms to raise or lower (this is the classic "cheat" by recruiting biceps or triceps)
- This is a small, concentrated movement, using very small muscles—so keep ROM small

VARIATIONS & PEEL BACKS
- **Variation:** *Kneeling* (Intermediate) (see page 129)

IMAGINE... *your arm emanates from your scapula.*

ELLIE SAYS... *"This is a great exercise for clients with sloping shoulders."*

MACHINE SET UP
- springs: 1 blue or 1 red
- bar: down
- ropes: standard length
- risers: down
- headrest: N/A

FUNCTIONS & TARGET MUSCLES
- Teaches Serape (serratus anterior connection to external obliques)
- Strengthens serratus anterior and anterior deltoid
- Peel back for *Balance Point* and *Teaser* (teaches *Teaser* arms)

ALIGNMENT CUES & OBSTACLES
- Do not let shoulders rise as your arms lift
- Do not lean back to lift arms, use abs to stabilize rib cage
- Keep pecs as relaxed as possible—widen arms if necessary

VARIATIONS AND PEEL BACKS
- **Variation:** *The Fairy* (Intermediate): Bring feet up and onto the front edge of the box, curve the lumbar spine without rounding the upper back (like *Coccyx Curl*), maintain the position while raising and lower arms from *Queen* exercise, keeping collarbones wide and shoulders away from ears

IMAGINE...*you are a queen lifting up heavy piles of gold dust—using your back to lift.*

SUSI SAYS...*"This motion makes me think of promo photos for the musical 'Evita,' so I like to sing, 'Don't cry for me Argentina'."*

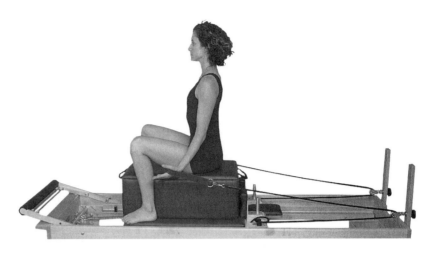

1. Starting Position—*4 repetitions*
Sit facing front of machine with legs on either side of box, feet flat on carriage, knees at 90˚, hands in loops with elbows slightly rounded and palms up. Arms are placed even with sides of the body.

Inhale and lengthen spine

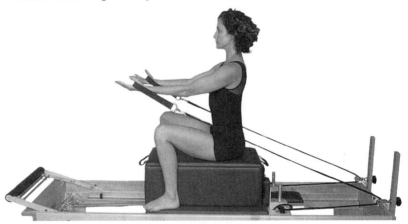

2. Exhale
Stabilize torso by pulling abdominals to spine. Think: down to go up. Shoulders pull down the back as arms lift to shoulder height.

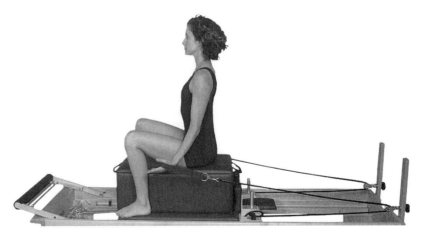

3. Inhale
Lengthen spine while lowering arms to Starting Position at hips.

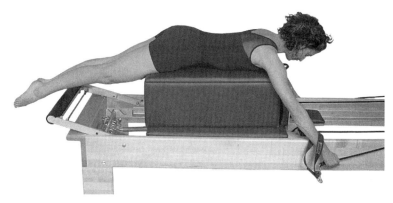

1. Starting Position—*5 repetitions*

Slide hands through loops and hold ropes just above D-ring. Keep spine neutral with head over headrest. Arms are straight and outside Reformer. Legs are straight with feet in Pilates "V". Use a small pillow between ankles, if necessary.

Inhale into back of ribs and lengthen spine to prepare

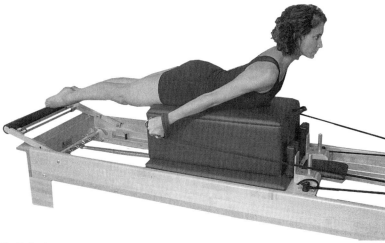

2. Exhale

Stabilize lumbar spine with low abdominals and low glutes and pull arms even with torso while upper thoracic spine reaches into extension; shoulders externally rotate, and collarbone widens as scapulae slide down the back.

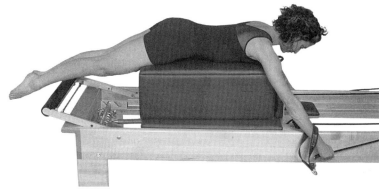

3. Inhale

Control carriage back to Starting Position while lowering head and upper body.

MACHINE SET UP
- springs: 1 blue or red
- bar: down
- ropes: standard length
- risers: down
- headrest: N/A

FUNCTIONS & TARGET MUSCLES
- Strengthens upper back extensors, posterior deltoids, lats, and lower traps
- Works sense of Neutral Spine while in a prone position
- Teaches upper back extension with shoulder stabilization

ALIGNMENT CUES & OBSTACLES
- Do not shorten back of neck—initiate extension from between scapulae, not top of head
- Keep elbows straight
- Place hands on client's calves to cue hip extensors, or place hand on low abdominals and cue small amount of lumbar flexion
- Place hyper-lordotic clients farther back on box so legs can be significantly lower than pelvis, or use a pillow under pelvis to facilitate slight lumbar flexion

VARIATIONS & PEEL BACKS
- **Modification:** If client is weak in upper back, use one blue spring
- **Variation:** To challenge client's coordination and make exercise advanced, add legs from *Swimming* exercise
- **Peel Backs:** *Lat Pull, Chest Expansion, Swan*

IMAGINE...*that the front of your shoulders are smiling open.*

ELLIE SAYS..."*This is a great exercise to re-train shoulder alignment to work the ever so important lower traps.*"

MACHINE SET UP

- springs: 1 blue or red
- bar: down
- ropes: standard length
- risers: down
- headrest: N/A

FUNCTIONS & TARGET MUSCLES

- Strengthens upper back extensors, infraspinatus, and posterior deltoids
- Teaches upper back extension with shoulder stabilization

ALIGNMENT CUES & OBSTACLES

- Through arm motion, pinky finger remains closest to body to avoid internal rotation of humerus
- Do not over-extend cervical spine
- Place hands on client's calves to cue hip extensors, or place hand on low abdominals to cue small amount of lumbar flexion
- Place hyper-lordotic clients farther back on box so legs can be significantly lower than pelvis, or use a pillow under pelvis to facilitate slight lumbar flexion
- Arms stay parallel to floor

VARIATIONS & PEEL BACKS

- **Modification:** If client has weak upper back, use one blue spring
- **Variation:** To challenge client's coordination and make exercise more advanced, combine *Charlie Chaplin* legs with this exercise
- **Peel Backs:** *Angels, Pulling Ropes*

IMAGINE...*that your hands are gliding over a table, sweeping off the crumbs.*

ELLIE SAYS...*"This is a prone Angel—much harder to stabilize your shoulders when you're on your belly!"*

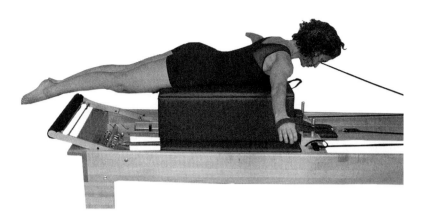

1. Starting Position—*5 repetitions*
Spine in neutral, arms open to sides with hands in line with shoulders making a "T," hands through loops with palms down. Upper back is held in slight extension. Legs are straight with feet in Pilates "V".

Inhale into back of ribs and lengthen spine to prepare

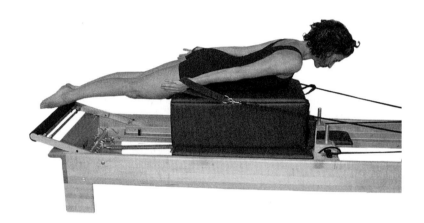

2. Exhale
Pull abdominals toward spine and pull arms to sides of torso, keeping elbows straight, arms parallel to floor, and palms down. Maintain slight upper back extension throughout exercise, but do not come up any higher than Starting Position.

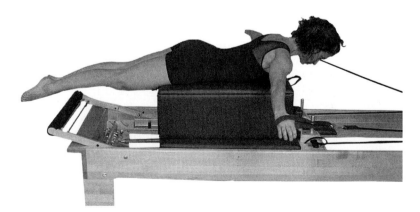

3. Inhale
Keeping upper spine in extension, control carriage back to Starting Position. Carriage should not hit home.

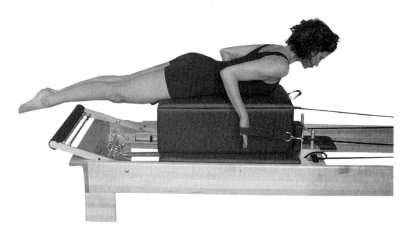

1. Starting Position—*8 repetitions*
Upper back in slight extension, hands in loops with elbows bent to 90°, fingertips toward floor, and upper arm glued to sides. Legs are straight with feet in Pilates "V". Pelvis is neutral.

Inhale into back of ribs and lengthen spine to prepare

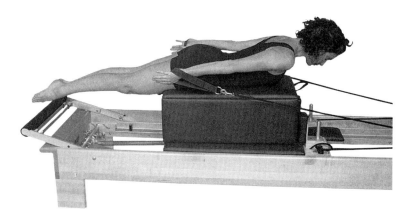

2. Exhale
Pull abdominals toward spine, straightening elbow while scapulae slide down back, keeping collarbones wide.

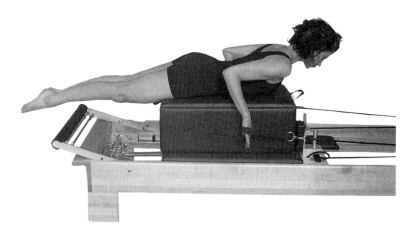

3. Inhale
Return forearm to Starting Position while maintaining shape and position of the torso.

MACHINE SET UP
- springs: 1 blue, 1 red or more for a challenge
- bar: down
- ropes: standard length
- risers: down
- headrest: N/A

FUNCTIONS & TARGET MUSCLES
- Strengthens triceps
- Strengthens upper back extensors

ALIGNMENT CUES & OBSTACLES
- Do not allow upper arm to lower or shoulders to internally rotate
- Do not snap elbows straight—lengthen the arms
- Keep upper arms parallel to floor
- Squeeze scapulae together to focus work on triceps
- Do not crunch back of neck

VARIATIONS & PEEL BACKS
- **Modification:** If client is weak use blue spring
- **Variation:** *Tricep Pulses*: keep arms straight and pulse palms up toward sky ten times
- **Peel Backs:** *Supine Triceps, Pulling Ropes*

ELLIE SAYS... *"These three prone arm exercises really help clients with forward head position. But the trainer must teach them to find extension in their thoracic spine, not just the top of their neck."*

BACKSTROKE

MACHINE SET UP
- springs: 1 or 2 red
- bar: down
- ropes: standard length
- risers: down
- headrest: N/A

FUNCTIONS & TARGET MUSCLES
- Strengthens abdominals, specifically the hard to find/work mid-abdominals
- Works deep neck flexors, hip flexors, lats, adductors, and serratus anterior
- Reinforces the Serape concept

ALIGNMENT CUES & OBSTACLES
- Perform this exercise smoothly with control and finesse—no jerking
- Keep pathway of arms and legs narrow—arm and leg movements mirror each other
- Legs and arms never drop below box—do not rely on momentum
- Ending "banana position" is two vertebrae higher than the Pilates Abdominal Position
- Even though rectus abdominis is working, make sure the transversus is pulling deeply to spine—no rectus "popping"
- Imprint lumbar spine into box for entire exercise (super scoop)
- **Obstacle:** Flat thoracic spine
- **Contraindications:** disc dysfunction, osteoporosis

VARIATIONS & PEEL BACKS
- Optional Stretch: After completing 4 repetitions, relax and open front of body—place feet on lowered footbar, arms dangle below box, and neck drapes over back edge of box
- **Advanced Variation:** Perform exercise in reverse order, going from Starting Position into "banana" shape, holding the shape for as long as possible as legs move apart, around, up and in.

IMAGINE...*you are performing water ballet, and the imaginary water provides resistance to control the movement of your limbs.*

DANO SAYS...*"I call this exercise 'The Patriotic Banana'."*

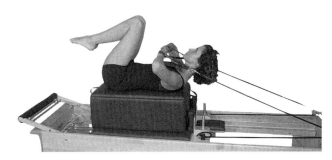

1. Starting Position—*4 repetitions*
Entire back of torso on long box with neck in deep flexion (hold that tangerine!), hands through loops placed just below chin in *Salute* position. Legs are in Table Top position with toes pointed.

Inhale to prepare

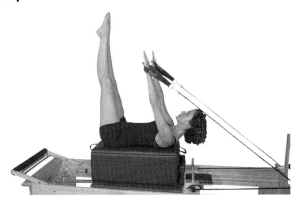

2. Exhale
Keeping upper back wide, reach fingers and toes to ceiling, making right angles at hips and shoulders. Keep legs touching, squeezing inner thighs together. Keep upper back wide and scapulae connected to box.

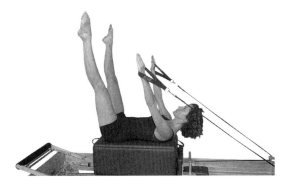

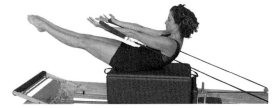

3. Breathing Continuously
Inhale as you open arms and legs. Exhale, externally rotate hips and shoulders to circle arms and legs forward and down while rolling spine up to "banana boat" position. Palms are up with fingers reaching away, heels are together in Pilates "V" Hold this elegant shape for another breath and as you slowly exhale all air remaining in your lungs, deeply imprint abdominals, reach your shoulders forward as you pull your sternum back. This really works the serratus anterior and helps stretch and round the thoracic spine. Inhale. Return to Starting Position.

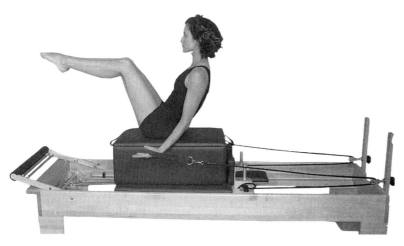

1. Starting Position—*4 repetitions*
Sitting in the middle of the box, just behind sit bones with lumbar spine in flexion. Hands are in loops and at hips, with palms up and elbows slightly bent. Raise legs one at time into Table Top position. You are now in the *Balance Point*.

Inhale to prepare

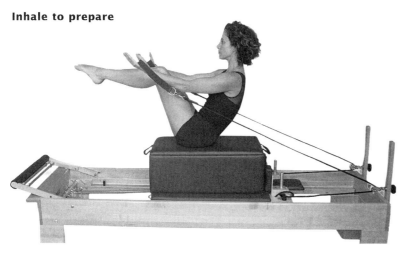

2. Exhale
Pull abdominals to spine and shoulders down the back as you reach arms up to shoulder height while maintaining *Balance Point* position (reach arms from hips to shoulders). Here's your Serape concept at work, back connecting to front.

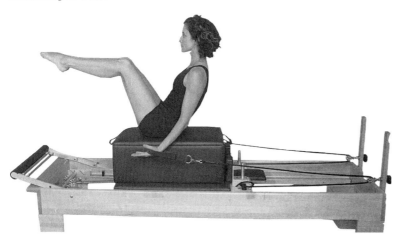

3. Inhale
Maintain abdominal connection and leg position while lowering arms to Starting Position at hips.

MACHINE SET UP
- springs: 1 red or 1 blue
- bar: down
- ropes: standard length
- risers: down
- headrest: N/A

FUNCTIONS & TARGET MUSCLES
- Works abdominals to maintain balance
- Works shoulder flexors and shoulder girdle stabilizers
- Works hip flexors
- Trains balance and coordination

ALIGNMENT CUES & OBSTACLES
- Do not let arms go behind torso—Range of Motion of arms is from hips to shoulders
- Practice *Queen* arms in *Balance Point* position on mat before adding spring resistance and carriage motion (this helps client feel secure performing exercise)
- Place hand just behind client's back to prevent client from falling
- Focus on anterior deltoid raising arm into to flexion so pec major doesn't overwork and round the upper back
- Before getting into *Balance Point* position, tell client to lower feet to box if they're about to fall
- **Contraindications:** disc dysfunction, osteoporosis

VARIATIONS & PEEL BACKS
- **Variation:** After performing 3 repetitions of exercise, raise arms and make 3 small arm circles, initiating movement from the scapulae. Lower arms. Raise arms and repeat circles reversing direction
- **Peel Backs:** *Queen, Fairy*

IMAGINE...*nothing is moving but your arms.*

ELLIE SAYS...*"Balance Point exemplifies the abdominals and Serape connection. Basically, if you're not working your back with your abdominals, you're going to fall."*

MACHINE SET UP
- springs: 1 red or 1 blue
- bar: down
- ropes: standard length
- risers: down
- headrest: N/A

FUNCTIONS & TARGET MUSCLES
- Strengthens abdominals and hip flexors
- Works lats, inner thighs, low glutes, and deep neck flexors

ALIGNMENT CUES & OBSTACLES
- Remember to use *Queen* arms—ROM from hips to shoulders
- Don't straighten lumbar spine when you reach *Balance Point* position at the top of the *Teaser*—keep that super scoop engaged
- Don't cheat and use momentum—remember control
- Keep shoulders away from ears—focus on using your Serape
- Feel energy emanating from belly button and extending out though hands and feet as body folds in half
- Make sure pelvis is not at front edge of box—this will feel precarious at top of *Teaser*
- **Obstacles:** Weak abdominals, weak hip flexors, tight hamstrings
- **Contraindications:** disc dysfunction, osteoporosis, neck or cervical injuries

VARIATIONS & PEEL BACKS
- **Peel Backs:** *Reverse Teaser, Queen, Balance Point, Roll Up* on Cadillac

IMAGINE...*folding your body in half around the center crease of your navel.*

ELLIE SAYS...*"The Teaser puts it all together: abdominal strength, Serape, sequential movement of the spine, balance, control and flexibility. Approach it with determination tempered with a sense of humor. Remember, laughing is good for the abdominals."*

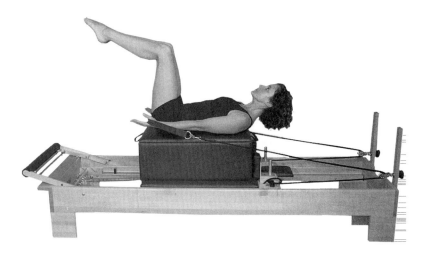

1. Starting Position—*3 repetitions with Arm Reaches, Circles, and Reverse Arm Circles*
Lie with back on box and legs in Table Top position, with arms out to sides and hands in loops, pulled into resistance.

Inhale to prepare

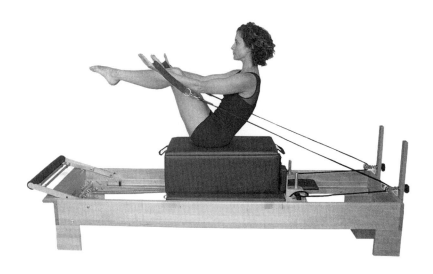

2. Exhale
Pull arms to sides, then reach hands towards knees and roll up sequentially through spine to *Balance Point* position, without lowering legs or losing Table Top position.

Lower arms to hip level and exhale to reach back up to shoulder level; repeat arm reach 3 times, repeating breathing sequence. After the 3rd reach, inhale and hold, then exhale and roll down one vertebra at a time while maintaining Table Top legs in the *Teaser* position.

Repeat two more times, on second repetition circle arms at the height of the shoulders, on the third repetition reverse the arm circles.

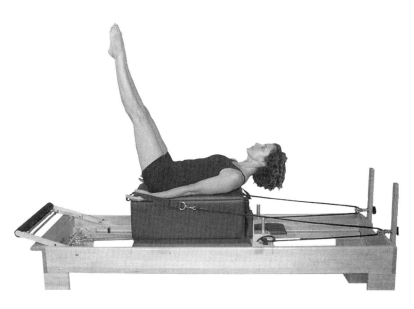

ADVANCED VARIATION: Legs Straight

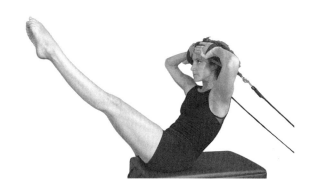

SUPER ADVANCED VARIATION: Salute 1

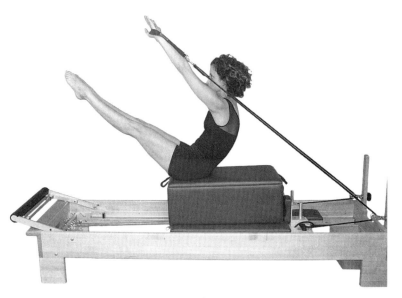

SUPER ADVANCED VARIATION: Salute 2

ADVANCED VARIATION:
Legs Straight
Same as Intermediate but keep legs straight in Pilates First Position the whole time.

SUPER ADVANCED VARIATION:
Salute
At top of *Teaser,* reach arms above head and bend elbows, bringing arms into *Salute* position (index fingers to eyebrows). Roll slightly forward of your *Balance Point* position while "saluting" arms out 3 times—keep shoulders down. You may want to lighten resistance to a blue spring.

MACHINE SET UP
- springs: 1 red or 1 blue
- bar: down
- ropes: standard length
- risers: down
- headrest: N/A

FUNCTIONS & TARGET MUSCLES
- Strengthens abdominals and hip flexors
- Works lats, inner thighs, low glutes, and deep neck flexors

ALIGNMENT CUES & OBSTACLES
- Remember to use *Queen* arms—ROM from hips to shoulders
- Don't straighten lumbar spine when you reach *Balance Point* position at the top of the *Teaser*—keep that super scoop engaged
- Don't cheat and use momentum—remember control
- Keep shoulders away from ears—focus on using your Serape
- Feel energy emanating from belly button and extending out though hands and feet as body folds in half
- Make sure pelvis is not at front edge of box—this will feel precarious at top of *Teaser*
- **Obstacles:** Weak abdominals, weak hip flexors, tight hamstrings
- **Contraindications:** disc dysfunction, osteoporosis, neck or cervical injuries

VARIATIONS & PEEL BACKS
- **Peel Backs:** *Advanced Teaser, Queen, Balance Point, Roll Up* on Cadillac

IMAGINE... *you are moving from your abdominals—not your hip flexors.*

ELLIE SAYS... *"This may be easier than the 'advanced version'—since it's easy to lever up from the hip flexors in Dead Hang."*

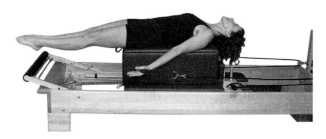

1. Starting Position—*3 repetitions*
Lying in *Dead Hang* position with back on box, scapulae just off back edge of box. Arms out to sides, with hands in loops pulling slightly into resistance. Legs are in Pilates First Position, hanging down slightly over front edge of box, head draped over back edge.

Inhale to prepare

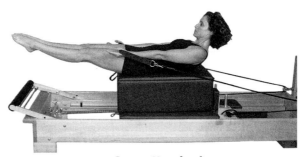

Super Hundred

2. Exhale/Inhale/Exhale
Exhale as you deepen abdominal engagement, squeeze low glutes, squeeze inner thighs together and roll up into *Super Hundred*. Inhale to hold then exhale up to the full *Teaser*, reaching arms to shoulder height.

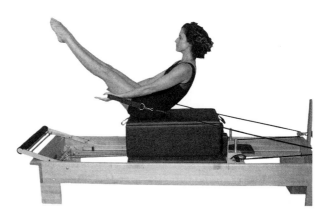

3. Breathing Continuously
Lower arms to hip level and exhale to reach back up to shoulder level; repeat arm reach 3 times, repeating breathing sequence. After the 3rd reach, inhale and hold, then exhale and roll down one vertebra at a time while maintaining legs in the *Teaser* position. Once you have imprinted your low back into onto the mat, lower legs to the *Super Hundred* position. Inhale for a moment holding the shape, then exhale and continue rolling down into Starting Position/*Dead Hang* (carriage does not go home).

Repeat the whole sequence again but at the top of the *Teaser*, circle arms 3 times in one direction, keeping at the height of the shoulders, then descend to *Dead Hang*. On the 3rd repetition, circle arms 3 times the opposite direction dead then descend to *Dead Hang*.

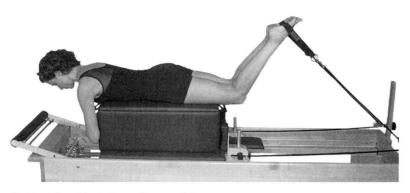

1. Starting Position—*8 repetitions*

Lying on stomach with knees just off back edge of box. Head is toward footbar with hands on front of box. Feet are pointed with loops around arches. Pubic bone pressed into carriage to keep lumbar spine long. For Parallel: inner thighs, knees, and ankles are touching. Knees are bent to about 60˚.

Inhale to prepare

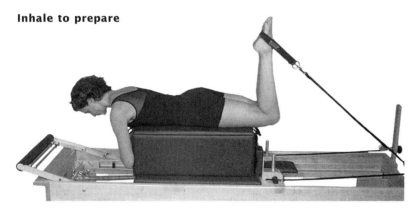

2–3. Exhale/Inhale

Pull abdominals to spine and tuck pelvis under, engaging glutes and pressing pubic bone into to box, while pulling feet towards glutes. Can initiate movement with a little push using hands. Knees bend to slightly past 90˚. Inhale. Keep abdominals working and control legs back to Starting Position.

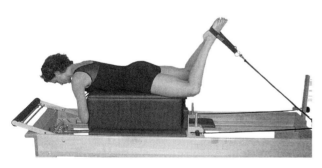

VARIATION: Turn Out

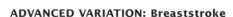

ADVANCED VARIATION: Breaststroke

MACHINE SET UP
- springs: 1 red, 1 blue, or 1 yellow
- bar: down
- ropes: to headrest or shorter
- risers: up or down
- headrest: N/A

FUNCTIONS & TARGET MUSCLES
- Strengthens hip extensors: hamstrings, and glutes
- In *Parallel*—works adductors
- In *Turn Out*—works external hip rotators

ALIGNMENT CUES & OBSTACLES
- Even though you're on your belly, keep abdominals engaged
- For clients with unstable knees—start with light springs and small ROM
- Stretch hamstrings after performing this exercise, or before, if client's hamstrings tend to cramp
- Assist the movement with hands on frame of Reformer—this will allow for more reps and less cramping

VARIATIONS & PEEL BACKS
- Can use ankle straps instead of loops, especially if feet tend to cramp
- **Variation:** *Single Leg*: Work one leg at a time using a lighter spring setting (not shown)
- **Variation:** *Medial Rotation:* brings knees together and feet apart to work medial hamstrings (good for postural knock knees and lateral rotation of the femurs)
- **Variation:** *Turn Out*: knees bent and opened wide off the edges of the box, with hips externally rotated, and heels touching
- **Variation:** *Breast Stroke In Turn Out* (Advanced): Add upper back extension with exaggerated breaststroke arms while legs pull toward glutes—body is folding in half backwards, focusing on abdominal and scapular engagement. Lower upper body when lowering legs

IMAGINE... *your pubic bone is glued down to the long box—no arching your back!*

ELLIE SAYS... *"The advanced variation is a killer for your butt, hamstrings, and back muscles."*

MACHINE SET UP
- springs: all
- bar: down
- ropes: N/A
- risers: N/A
- headrest: N/A

FUNCTIONS & TARGET MUSCLES
- Strengthens hip extensors: hamstrings, and glutes
- Works deep six lateral hip rotators
- Works inner thighs

ALIGNMENT CUES & OBSTACLES
- Initiate motion from upper inner thigh, rather than heels
- Keep abdominals scooped to protect lumbar spine
- Keep the beats small and precise—open legs no further than width of hips
- To avoid working lumbar spine extensors, slide hip crease to back edge of box and keep heels lower than pelvis

VARIATIONS & PEEL BACKS
- **Variation:** Lower legs for 4 heel beats, then raise them for 4 beats—repeat for 5 sets
- **Variation:** Place accent on the out motion to work hip abductors
- **Variation:** *Scissors* are like a "changement" in ballet: alternately cross your heels as you count up for 4 and down for 4

IMAGINE......*there's no place like home.*

ELLIE SAYS.....*"Everyone loves a good butt exercise."*

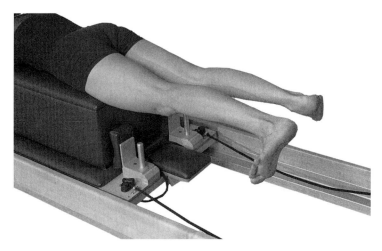

1. Starting Position—*20 repetitions*
Lying prone on box with head at front end of Reformer and hip crease close to back edge of box. Hips in external rotation with knees straight and feet flexed. Hold onto front of box, head down. Shoulders stay relaxed.

Inhale to prepare

2. Breathing Continuously
Keeping knees straight and feet flexed, open and close legs, lightly clapping heels together. Place accent on "in" motion of legs. Continue to beat heels together, deepening abdominal engagement with every exhalation.

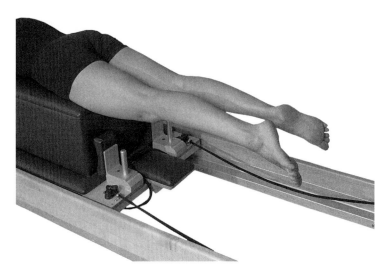

3. Breathing Continuously
Repeat with pointed feet.

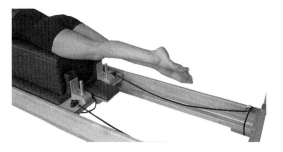

VARIATION: Scissors

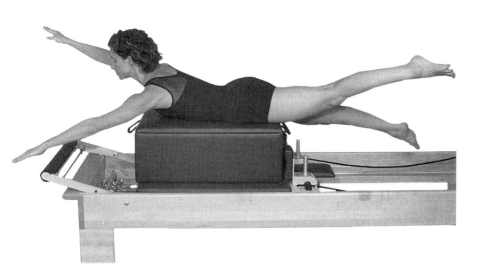

1. Starting Position—*3 or 4 sets of ten*
Lying prone on box with head at front end of Reformer and hip crease close to back edge of box. Arms straight by the ears and at least shoulder width apart. Legs straight with hips in slight external rotation.

Inhale to prepare

2. Breathing Continuously
Raise upper back and head into extension, gazing onto lowered footbar. Slide shoulder blades down back and pull abdominals to spine. Raise right leg and left arm about 1–2", then alternate. Begin with slow, small motions and increase speed and Range of Motion as strength and ability allow.

Continue breathing continuously, deepening abdominal engagement and sliding scapulae down back with every exhalation.

MACHINE SET UP
- springs: all
- bar: down
- ropes: N/A
- risers: N/A
- headrest: N/A

FUNCTIONS & TARGET MUSCLES
- Strengthens glutes, hamstrings, and back extensors
- Teaches contralateral patterning in prone position
- Works mid and low traps, abdominals, and multifidi

ALIGNMENT CUES & OBSTACLES
- When raising arm and opposite leg, reach scapula and opposite hip towards one another to prevent pelvis from rocking side to side
- If client is over using lumbar extensors, cue low abdominals by sliding hand under client's belly
- If client is extremely lordodic, keep lumbar in small amount of flexion by placing heels lower than pelvis, and/or cue client to press pubic bone into box
- Widen arms and allow elbows to soften if upper traps are overly engaged/tight or if lats are too tight
- Lifting the legs higher works the glutes more (but don't hyperextend lumbar spine to raise legs)
- Move slowly at first to really emphasize movement pattern and glute engagement

VARIATIONS & PEEL BACKS
- **Modification:** Start with lifting just one arm and opposite leg, holding the footbar for support. This is a great way to train contralateral movement. When client is stronger, try the full *Swimming*
- **Modification:** *Swimming Legs*: Keeping head down, holding front of box, tuck pelvis under by scooping belly in and squeezing glutes, and do small *Swimming* kicks keeping pelvis and spine stable

IMAGINE...*a shark is chasing you in the ocean.*

SUSI SAYS...*"It is so important to work the spine in slight extension since so much of Pilates is in flexion."*

ROCKING SWAN

MACHINE SET UP
- springs: all
- bar: down
- ropes: N/A
- risers: N/A
- headrest: N/A

FUNCTIONS & TARGET MUSCLES
- Strengthens back extensors
- Works shoulder stabilizers, triceps, and abdominals
- Stretches rectus abdominis

ALIGNMENT CUES & OBSTACLES
- Maintain the arc of the body while elbows bend
- Do not crunch back of neck
- Bend elbows in toward body, not out to the sides
- Do not hyperextend elbows when straightening arms
- On *High Swan*, really scoop belly in
- Put a ball between ankles for more glute and inner thigh work
- **Contraindications:** Low back injuries (due to extreme spinal extension)

VARIATIONS & PEEL BACKS
- **Peel Backs:** *Swan* on Cadillac and Wunda Chair, *Swan Dive* on Mat

IMAGINE...*your body is a seesaw and your pelvis is the fulcrum.*

SUSI SAYS...*"Think of the Rocking Swan as the inverse of Rolling Like A Ball. It's about maintaining the shape of the body while moving that shape up and down, or around. They're complementary exercises."*

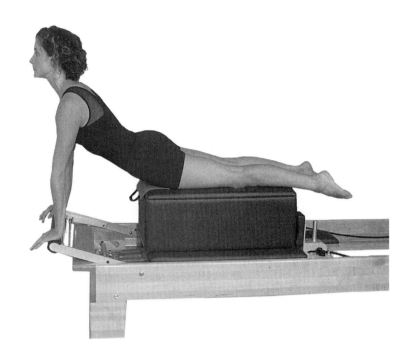

1. Starting Position—*3 repetitions*
In *Swan* position (entire spine is in extension) facing front of Reformer with hands on footbar shoulder width apart, legs and pelvis on box. Legs are open slightly wider than hips, hips are externally rotated, glutes are engaged, and feet are pointed.

Inhale to lengthen spine

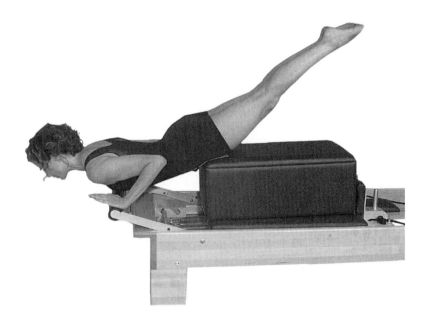

2–3. Exhale/Inhale
Pull abdominals to spine, slide shoulders down back, engage low glutes and maintain *Swan* position while bending elbows. Legs lift as you descend, staying in one piece. Inhale. Return to Starting Position by straightening elbows, which brings legs and pelvis back onto box.

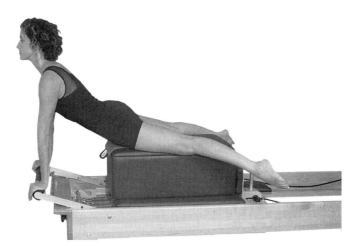

1. Starting Position—*3 repetitions*

In *Swan* position (entire spine is in extension) facing front of Reformer with hands on footbar shoulder width apart, legs and pelvis on box. Legs are open shoulder width, hips are externally rotated, glutes are engaged, and feet are pointed.

Inhale to lengthen spine

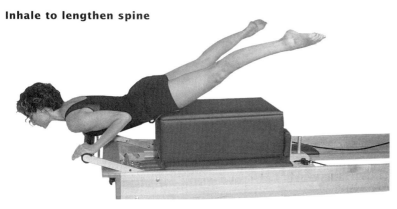

2. Exhale

Pull abdominals to spine, slide shoulders down back, engage low glutes and maintain *Swan* position while bending elbows. Legs lift as you descend, staying in one piece.

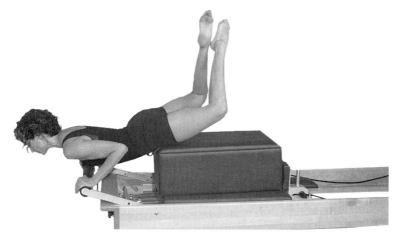

3. Breathing Continuously

When elbows are bent and pelvis is suspended above the box, slightly bend knees and criss-cross ankles by moving legs open and close from the hip joint, not the knee.

After 8 repetitions, straighten knees, then straighten elbows, returning to Starting Position.

MACHINE SET UP
- springs: all
- bar: down
- ropes: N/A
- risers: N/A
- headrest: N/A

FUNCTIONS & TARGET MUSCLES
- Strengthens back extensors
- Works shoulder stabilizers, triceps, and abdominals
- Strengthens external rotators of the hip
- Stretches rectus abdominis

ALIGNMENT CUES & OBSTACLES
- Maintain shape of leg and angle of knee while opening and closing legs from hip joint
- Maintain the arc of the body while elbows bend
- Do not crunch back of neck
- Bend elbows in toward body, not out to the sides
- Do not hyperextend elbows when straightening arms
- On *High Swan*, really scoop belly in
- Put a ball between ankles for more glute and inner thigh work
- **Contraindications:** Low back injuries (due to extreme spinal extension)

VARIATIONS & PEEL BACKS
- **Peel Backs:** *Rocking Swan*

IMAGINE...*your legs lift up toward the sky with your glutes—not your lower back.*

ELLIE SAYS...*"Add a quick changement as you rise up out of the Grasshopper for more fun."*

roll down series

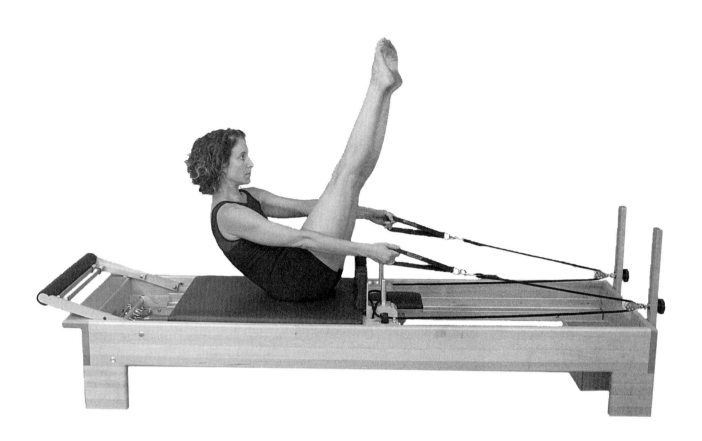

The Roll Down Series is perfectly placed after the extension exercises on the Long Box. Always remember that it feels really good to do flexion exercises after extension. Seated flexion is contraindicated for disc dysfunction, osteoporosis, and SI joint instability. The ropes are shortened to top of headrest to provide extra resistance or help. Don't forget to lengthen ropes back to standard length after completing the Roll Down Series.

ROLL DOWNS	**REVERSE TEASERS**
with Bicep Curls	*Table Top Legs*
with Rhomboids	*Legs Straight*
	Can-Can
	Bent to Straight

MACHINE SET UP

- springs: 1 red & 1 blue
- bar: down
- ropes: shortened with loops to top of headrest
- risers: down
- headrest: down, with sticky pad

FUNCTIONS & TARGET MUSCLES

- Strengthens abdominals
- Reinforces sequential movement of the spine
- Stretches deep muscles of spine
- Teaches shoulder girdle stabilization

ALIGNMENT CUES & OBSTACLES

- Feel spine lengthening even as it is curving—spine does not compress into flexion
- When rolling up keep elbows straight in order to focus work in the abdominals and prevent the biceps from assisting
- Avoid sinking into sternum to initiate *Roll Down*—this just increases forward head posture—start the action with a *Coccyx Curl*, lumbar C-Curve and low glute engagement
- Make the work happen from bottom of spine up—focus on Abdominal Scoop
- *Roll Downs* and variations should be smooth and controlled
- Feel free to stop client mid-way down if they are overusing rectus. Have them inhale without moving, then exhale re-engaging Abdominal Scoop ("navel to the spine") before continuing the *Roll Down*
- **Contraindications:** Coccyx injuries, disc dysfunction, osteoporosis, SI joint instability

VARIATIONS & PEEL BACKS

- Lighter spring resistance makes the exercise more difficult
- **Variation:** *Pearl Button Roll Down*: Start the *Roll Down* but stop once you've imprinted your sacrum onto the carriage. Inhale and hold, and on the exhale *Roll Down* one vertebra (*Pearl Button* on your imaginary cardigan). Inhale and hold, continue with your stop and start action until you've rolled down 5 *Pearl Buttons*. Continue with the *Roll Down* and repeat this sequence on the way up

IMAGINE...*your spine is a strand of pearls, which you place down and peel up one pearl at a time.*

ELLIE SAYS...*"This is the ultimate peel back for the Roll Up/Roll Down on the mat. Keep decreasing the resistance until you're on your own. Also, think of this as a stretch for your back muscles as much as an abdominal exercise."*

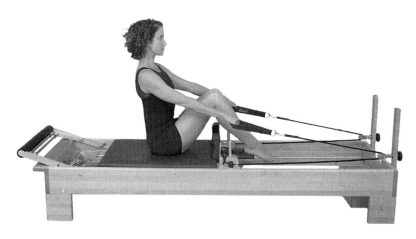

1. Starting Position—*3 to 5 repetitions*

Seated facing back of Reformer with arches at top of headrest. Hands in loops, elbows straight with palms facing toward body (shoulders in neutral). Seated on sit bones with spine straight. Scapulae are engaged down back, pulling carriage into resistance.

Inhale and feel the "golden string" lengthening the spine from the crown of your head

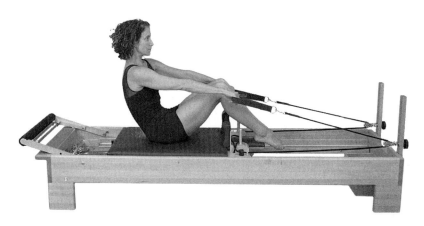

2. Exhale

Pull navel to spine and engage low glutes, initiating a C-Curve at the base of the spine. Articulate down one vertebra at a time, from bottom to top, until entire back is on carriage with head looking up at the sky (keep holding that tangerine between chin and chest).

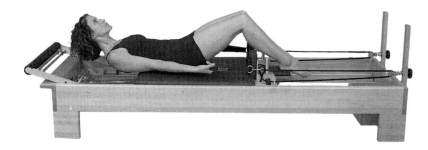

3. Inhale

Roll shoulders open until palms are facing upward, and widen the back. Maintain abdominal connection to spine.

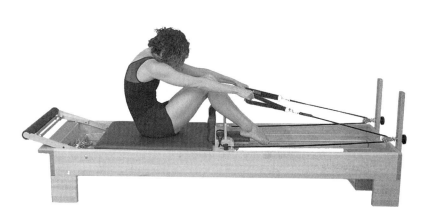

4. Exhale
Deepen low Abdominal Scoop and imprint low back onto carriage as you roll up one vertebra at a time, until seated on sit bones with entire spine in one large C-Curve.

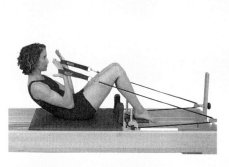

VARIATION: with Bicep Curls
(Beginning/Intermediate) *Roll Down* one third of the way. Inhale and rotate palms to ceiling. Perform *Bicep Curl* on exhale, maintaining torso level, and deepening Abdominal Scoop with each exhale. After 8 repetitions, continue *Roll Down.*

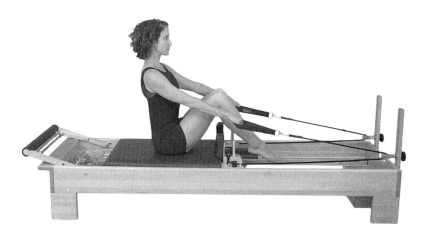

5. Inhale
Stack up the spine, returning to the Starting Position.

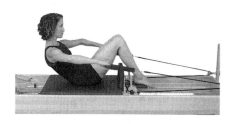

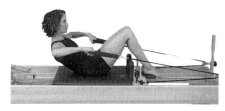

VARIATION: with Rhomboids
(Beginning/Intermediate) *Roll Down* one third of the way. Inhale while moving arms into *Rhomboid* position. Pull scapulae together on exhale, maintaining torso position at the same level and deepening Abdominal Scoop with each exhale. After 8 repetitions, continue *Roll Down.*

MACHINE SET UP

- springs: 1 red & 1 blue
- bar: down
- ropes: shortened with loops to top of headrest
- risers: down
- headrest: down

FUNCTIONS & TARGET MUSCLES

- Strengthens abdominals and hip flexors
- Reinforces sequential spinal movement
- Teaches shoulder girdle stabilization
- Peel back for all *Teaser* exercises

ALIGNMENT CUES & OBSTACLES

- Don't allow legs to drop while rolling up or down through spine
- Keep the motion smooth and steady to make sure the abdominals and hip flexors do the work, not momentum
- Do not lean back while straightening the legs into *Teaser* position—feel body folding in half
- Keep lumbar spine in small C-Curve while trying to extend upper back and neck
- **Obstacles:** Tight hamstrings and weak hip flexors
- **Contraindications:** disc dysfunction, osteoporosis, SI joint instability, coccyx injuries

VARIATIONS & PEEL BACKS

- **Peel Backs:** *Roll Downs, Balance Point*

IMAGINE...*someone or something is holding your thighs so they cannot move while torso rolls up and down.*

ELLIE SAYS...*"This is the easiest version of the Teaser. Master this and the Teaser will be yours (with some sweat and work)."*

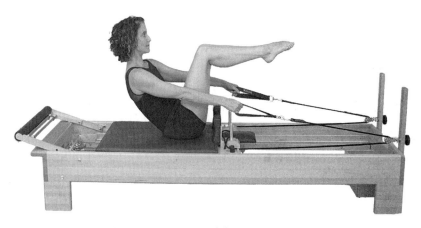

1. Starting Position—*3 to 5 repetitions*
Holding the loops, move pelvis as close as possible to shoulder rests, sit up in your *Balance Point*, lifting legs into Table Top position. Squeeze inner thighs together, arms extending in front of you at shoulder height, palms facing each other.

Inhale to prepare

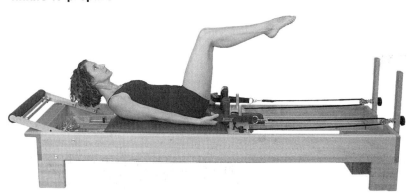

2. Exhale
Articulate down one vertebra at a time until you're lying on the carriage.

3. Inhale
Breathe into your back at the bottom.

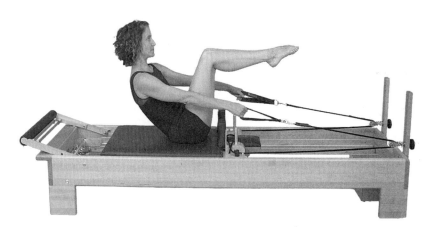

4. Exhale
Feel the scapulae pulling down the back as you Squeeze a Tangerine under your chin, and articulate up one vertebra at a time coming back up to your *Balance Point*. Maintain the Table Top Legs throughout, and keep squeezing those inner thighs together.

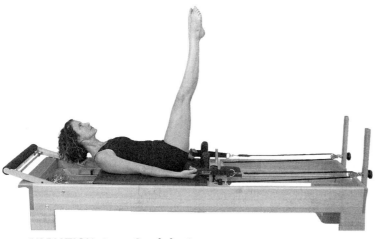

VARIATION: Legs Straight 1

INTERMEDIATE VARIATION:
Legs Bent to Straight
Straighten legs while rolling up into the *Teaser*, and bend knees into Table Top while rolling down (not shown).

ADVANCED VARIATION:
Legs Straight
Begin with straight legs and feet in Pilates "V" *Teaser* position, and keep legs straight throughout exercise—do not allow legs to lower or rise.

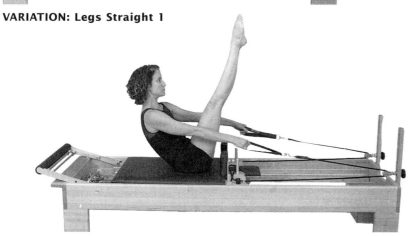

VARIATION: Legs Straight 2

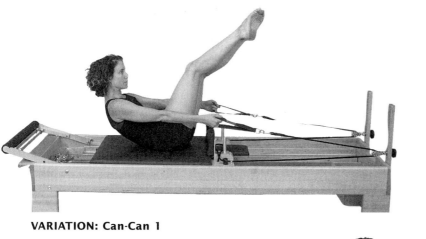

VARIATION: Can-Can 1

ADVANCED VARIATION: Can-Can
Keeping both sit bones on carriage, rotate Table Top Legs to right and articulate up on right side of spine. In *Teaser* position straighten legs, keeping legs on the right side of the body. Inhale and maintain position. Exhale, bend legs into Table Top, and roll down on right side of spine. Alternate sides and repeat for 3 sets.

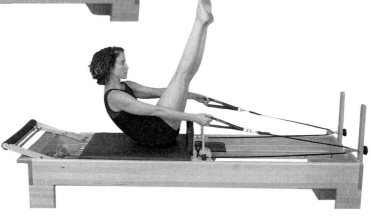

VARIATION: Can-Can 2

MERMAID

MACHINE SET UP
- springs: 1 red
- bar: high
- ropes: N/A
- risers: N/A
- headrest: N/A

FUNCTIONS & TARGET MUSCLES
- Stretches quadratus lumborum, internal and external obliques, lats, and pecs
- Teaches sequential spinal movement to the side
- Works spinal mobility in all planes of motion
- Strengthens triceps (during *Push Up* phase)

ALIGNMENT CUES & OBSTACLES
- ROM of lateral flexion/side bending is smaller toward internally rotated hip, so when stretching toward risers, reach out on diagonal more than bending side to avoid knee compression
- As always, keep scapulae stabilized and shoulders away from ears—push carriage out from armpit, not upper trap
- Keep abdominals engaged to lift torso up and out of pelvis—this helps to relax hips and decreases pressure on knees
- Remember that the neck is part of the spine—keep neck in line with curve of the spine when side bending
- **Obstacles:** Tight hips, tight back, tight shoulders
- **Contraindications:** Shoulder instability in *Carve a Sphere* and *Push Up* variations, knee injuries, arthritis of hip and/or knee, disc dysfunction, osteoporosis

VARIATIONS & PEEL BACKS
- If "Z" legs are uncomfortable or impossible—support internally rotated hip with pillow or mat beneath sit bone, or bend both knees together toward shoulder rests so side of hip rests on carriage
- **Peel Backs:** *Side Stretch* on Cadillac, *Mermaid* in Mat Series

IMAGINE...*you are a mermaid and your legs are your tail that you have swished to the side so you can stretch luxuriously on a warm rock in a tide pool.*

ELLIE SAYS...*"When you take the time to stretch your client open while they are Carving the Sphere, you'll see immediate results."*

SUSI SAYS...*"So much of Pilates is about stability. This is a mobility exercise for the back and shoulders. It's a wonderful stretch—enjoy it."*

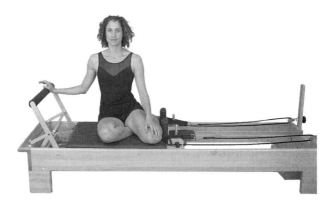

1. Starting Position—*3 repetitions each side*
Seated on Reformer facing the side. Legs folded into a "Z" shape with the leg closest to risers internally rotated, with knee bent and shin against the shoulder rests. The other leg is externally rotated with knee bent toward footbar and calf placed in front of the body. Sit on one hip. (This is 4th position in Graham Technique floor work.) Place heel of hand on footbar in line with ear.

Inhale, lengthen spine and reach arm from shoulder rest toward ceiling—keep shoulder down

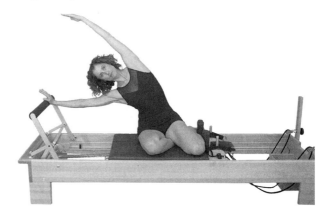

2-4. Breathing Continuously
Exhale, stabilize scapula and straighten elbow to push carriage away from home while side bending toward footbar, reaching opposite arm up and over to stretch. Inhale. Hold stretch, breathing into ribs, stretching the intercostals. Exhale. Return back to Starting Position.

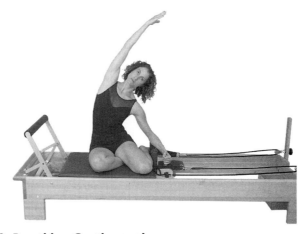

5-8. Breathing Continuously
Inhale to lengthen spine. Exhale as you reach opposite arm up to ceiling and side bend toward risers. Inhale. Hold stretch breathing into ribs to increase stretch. Exhale. Return to Starting Position moving sequentially from base of spine and lower arm to footbar, ready to repeat sequence.

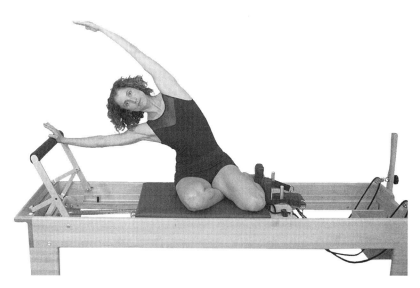

Spine Twist with Push Ups 1

Spine Twist with Push Ups
On second repetition, push elbow
to straight.

1. Exhale
Side bend halfway toward footbar, hollow
front of the body creating space to twist
both shoulders toward bar, placing hands
at corners of bar.

2. Inhale
Bend elbows high and wide bringing head
underneath (or for very tight shoulders,
over the footbar).

3. Exhale
Engage abdominals to push away from
footbar keeping torso low and scapulae
engaged. Repeat for 3–5 *Push Ups*.

Transition back to the Starting Position.

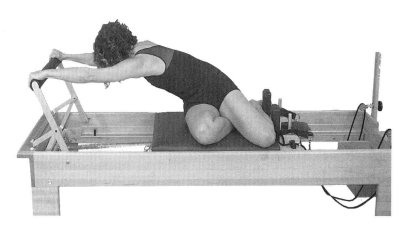

Spine Twist with Push Ups 2

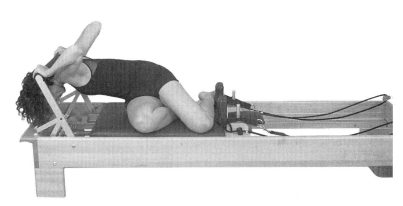

Spine Twist with Push Ups 3

MERMAID: CARVE A SPHERE

Carve a Sphere
On third repetition, when stretching toward risers make a HUGE arm circle with torso remaining bent to side.

1. Inhale
Begin by opening arm and chest toward ceiling. Maintain upper body rotation and extension while reaching and circling arm behind body, continue circling arm down toward side (really reach arm behind body to stretch pecs).

2. Exhale
Lower hand and brush past side of body to reach forward, pulling torso forward into flexion (resist motion with abdominals to stretch QL).

3. Inhale
Continue circling arm toward risers to complete the circle.

Reverse the direction of the circle, going from flexion to extension with upper body. After completing full circle, continue moving torso forward until it is centered, then stack up spine from bottom to top, ending in an upright, seated position.

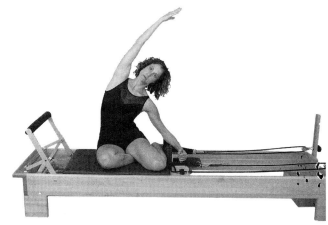

Carve a Sphere Starting Position

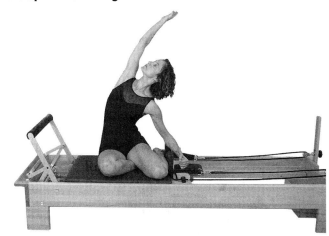

Carve a Sphere 1

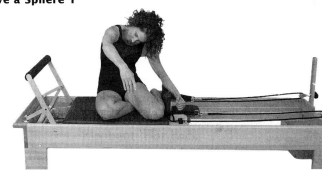

Carve a Sphere 2

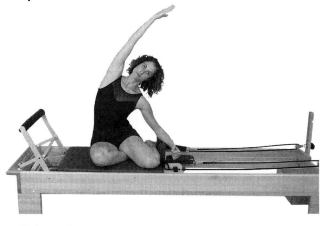

Carve a Sphere 3

plank/long stretch series

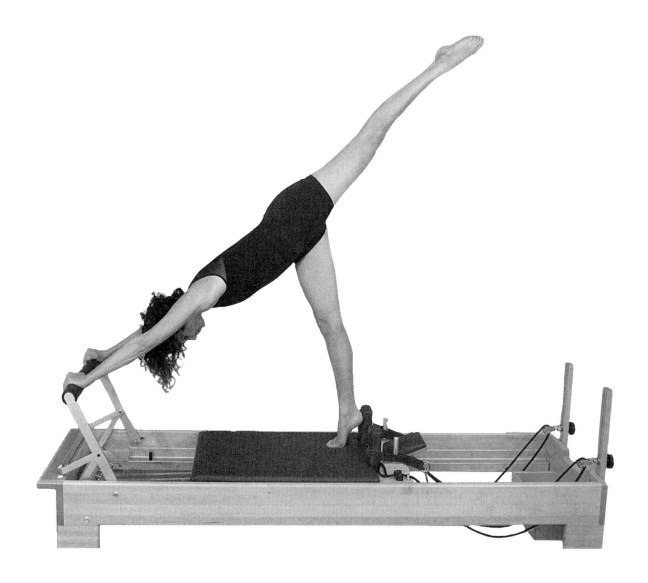

The exercises in the Plank Series are full body exercises, challenging the core, upper body, legs and butt. Exercises from this series should be incorporated into every workout since they efficiently train and challenge the body. This series can be hard on the wrists, so warm up the wrists with gentle circling before starting this series. If you are shorter than 5'5" you can modify the series by placing a roller in front of the shoulder rests. To increase core challenge, lighten springs or do the series in second gear.

BEGINNING	**INTERMEDIATE**	**ADVANCED**
Elephant	*Plank/Long Stretch*	*Down Stretch*
Forward Bend Stretch	*"U" Pull*	*Arabesque*
	Around the World/Up Stretch	*FTD Florist*
		Long Back Stretch

PLANK/LONG STRETCH

MACHINE SET UP
- springs: 1 red & 1 blue or yellow
- bar: high
- ropes: N/A
- risers: N/A
- headrest: up, with sticky pad

FUNCTIONS & TARGET MUSCLES
- Works pecs, serratus anterior, lats, abdominals, erectors, hamstrings, and glutes
- Strengthens shoulder stabilizers, emphasizing the serratus anterior to prevent scapular winging

ALIGNMENT CUES & OBSTACLES
- Getting onto the machine is part of the exercise (hand, hand, foot, foot). The carriage should not move as you do this— yep, you must use your abdominals
- Maintain *Plank* position—do not let pelvis sag down to floor or pike up toward ceiling
- Press through heels to engage hamstrings and glutes
- Keep fingers long and wrists straight to avoid compression
- Focus eyes toward floor to avoid crunching back of neck
- Try to bring carriage to home position with shoulders directly over wrists
- Do not hyperextend elbows
- Peel back for *Around the World, Control Front, Arabesque, Knee Stretch: Knees Off*
- **Contraindications:** Wrist problems, Carpal Tunnel Syndrome, or shoulder injuries

VARIATIONS & PEEL BACKS
- **Variation:** for a serious core challenge, try this exercise on 1 spring and have client take 5 counts to press out and 5 counts to come in!
- **Peel Backs:** *Flat Back Knee Stretches, Elephant, Plank* position and *Control Front* on the Mat

IMAGINE...*you are a solid board from the tip of your head to your reaching heels.*

ELLIE SAYS...*"Great stabilization exercises for those noodle-y people."*

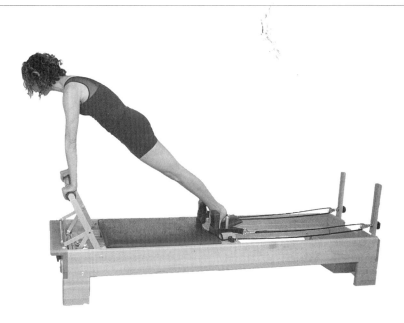

1. Starting Position—*4 repetitions*
Begin in a push up position with hands on footbar shoulder width apart and toes on headrest with heels together. Hollow upper back slightly, engaging serratus anterior, squeeze inner thighs, and engage hamstrings and glutes.

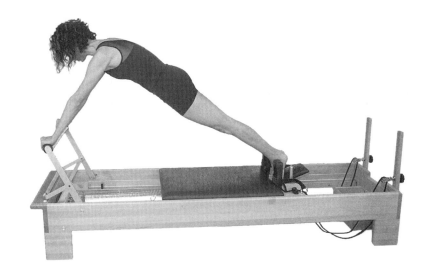

2. Inhale
Press carriage out as far as possible using arms; maintain shoulder stability and Neutral Spine/Pelvis.

3. Exhale
Pull abdominals to spine, squeeze heels together, and pull carriage home (or as close as possible) using lats. Maintain shoulder stability and Neutral Spine/Pelvis.

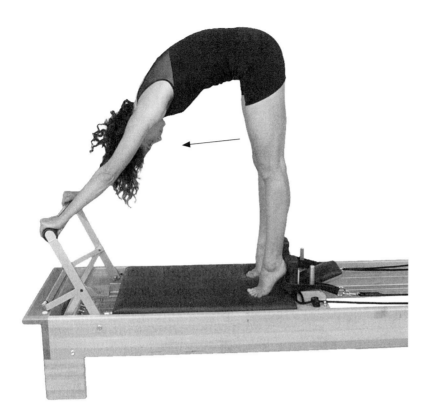

MACHINE SET UP
- springs: 1 red & 1 blue or yellow
- bar: high
- ropes: N/A
- risers: N/A
- headrest: N/A

FUNCTIONS & TARGET MUSCLES
- Teaches lower body movement initiated with spinal flexion
- Works abdominals and scapula stabilizers
- Challenges ankle stability
- Peel back for *Up Stretch* on Wunda Chair

ALIGNMENT CUES & OBSTACLES
- Stay out of upper traps as much as possible
- Don't let ankle joints roll out—clients can see their feet in this position, so point it out to them
- Poke client just above belly button and tell them to initiate from abdominals, not legs
- **Contraindications:** Disc dysfunction, shoulder problems, osteoporosis

VARIATIONS & PEEL BACKS
- **Peel Back:** *Round Back Knee Stretch*

IMAGINE…*a hot air balloon rising to the sky and pulling mid-back into flexion to move carriage -or- imagine you're making a "U" with your spine.*

SUSI SAYS…*"And today presenting the letter 'U'—you."*

1. Starting Position—*5 to 10 repetitions*
Hands on bar shoulder width apart or wider, with fingers reaching long and wrists as straight as possible. Heels against shoulder rests in relevé. Spine rounded as much as possible—focus on lumbar and lower thoracic spine curving.

2. Inhale
Push carriage out a few inches without moving shoulders.

3. Exhale
Pull abdominals to the sky to round the back; carriage should move toward home 3–5".

The *"U" Pull* is performed with relatively quick pulsing motions, pulling from the abdominals, accenting the "in" motion.

AROUND THE WORLD/UP STRETCH

MACHINE SET UP
- springs: 1 red & 1 blue or yellow
- bar: up
- ropes: N/A
- risers: N/A
- headrest: N/A

FUNCTIONS & TARGET MUSCLES
- Works pecs, serratus anterior, lats, abdominals, spinal extensors, hamstrings, and glutes
- Reinforces sequential movement of the spine

ALIGNMENT CUES & OBSTACLES
- The head is last body part to come into the *Plank* position
- Keep shoulders away from ears and do not overextend neck
- Use glutes, hamstrings, and abdominals to support *Plank* position
- Think of this exercise as a way to entertain the brain while working the arms
- **Contraindications:** Wrist problems, Carpal Tunnel Syndrome, shoulder injuries, osteoporosis

VARIATIONS & PEEL BACKS
- **Modification:** Prepare for motion by practicing moving from *"U" Pull* into *Plank* position and back to *"U" Pull*, thinking of the pelvis as the motor behind the movement
- **Variation:** For "extra credit" try reversing the motion—push out into *Plank*, move carriage toward home while snaking through spine from tail to head into *Plank* position over the bar, lengthen body into *Plank* and repeat
- **Peel Backs:** *"U" Pull, Plank*

IMAGINE...*your spine is a snake.*

SUSI SAYS...*"Break dancing meets Pilates— doing The Worm on the Reformer. Oh yeah."*

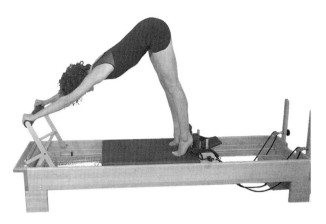

1. Starting Position—*4 repetitions*
Begin in "downward dog position" with hands on footbar shoulder width apart and feet in relevé with heels pressing into shoulder rests. Fold at the hips, dropping armpits down toward knees. The carriage may not stay home if you are tall.

Inhale into upper back to prepare

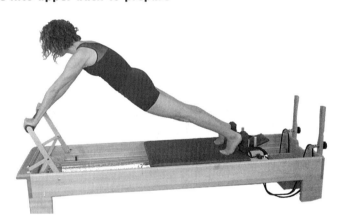

2. Exhale
Using hamstrings, push carriage away from home as far as possible. Keeping carriage still, lengthen spine into *Plank* position moving sequentially from pelvis to head. Spine should ripple like a wave.

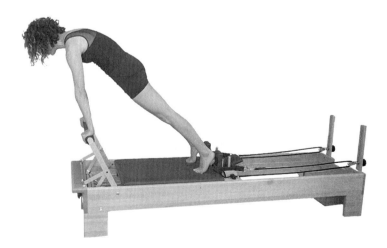

3. Inhale
Maintain *Plank* position and bring carriage all the way home. Pull abdominals to spine, rounding upper back from serratus, transitioning back to Starting Position.

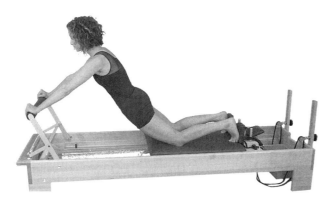

Transition
From *Plank* position of last repetition of *Around the World/Up Stretch,* place knees onto carriage and lower pelvis, extending entire spine to create one long curve from the knees to top of the head. Slide feet back to shoulder rests.

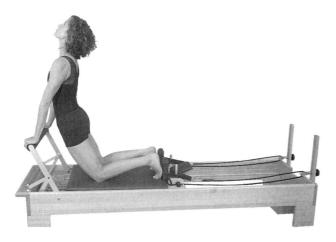

1. Starting Position—*4 repetitions*
Deepen abdominal connection to spine, engage glutes to protect low back and pull carriage home using arms, keep elbows straight and maintain the shape of the body. Allow sternum to reach to the ceiling, but don't crunch the neck by dropping the head backwards.

Inhale and lengthen spine

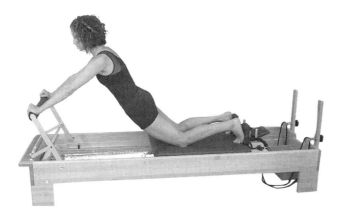

2. Exhale
Lengthen spine and push carriage out, maintaining your shape.

3. Inhale
Return to Starting Position. Lift chest and rise up, coming up to fingertips to finish.

MACHINE SET UP
- springs: 1 red & 1 blue or yellow
- bar: up
- ropes: N/A
- risers: N/A
- headrest: N/A

FUNCTIONS & TARGET MUSCLES
- Opens chest and works upper back extensors
- Works pecs, lats, abdominals, erectors, hamstrings, and glutes
- Stretches front of the body

ALIGNMENT CUES & OBSTACLES
- Even though abdominals are in a lengthened position, use them with glutes to feel torso lifting out of wrists
- Think of the body shape as the inverse of a C-Curve
- Stabilize scapulae and keep shoulders away from ears
- **Contraindications:** Wrist, shoulder, knee problems

VARIATIONS & PEEL BACKS
- Teaching Tool: When the carriage comes home on the first the repetition, maintain full body arch and peel hands from footbar so just the fingertips are touching—feel the torso lift off the knees and hands. Place hands back on footbar maintaining this lengthened and supported sensation throughout exercise
- **Peel Backs:** *Plank, Chest Expansion*

IMAGINE...*you're scraping the inside of a large tube with the front of your body.*

ELLIE SAYS...*"Great example of the Pilates powerhouse used in opposition to spinal extension."*

MACHINE SET UP

- springs: 1 red & 1 blue or yellow
- bar: high
- ropes: N/A
- risers: N/A
- headrest: N/A

FUNCTIONS & TARGET MUSCLES

- Strengthens glute max, hamstrings, and external rotators of the hips
- Works scapula stabilizers, abdominals, spinal extensors, and hip flexors
- Stretches hamstrings

ALIGNMENT CUES & OBSTACLES

- Turn out occurs at hip joint, not pelvis— keep pelvis square and work the "deep six" to externally rotate the femur in the air
- Emphasis is on the "up" motion of top leg— do not allow leg to drop
- Think of this *Arabesque* as the splits rotated 90˚
- Keep shoulders away from ears
- Don't crunch back of neck in effort to increase height of leg
- Do not lock or hyperextend knee of standing leg
- **Contraindications:** Tight hamstrings, tight lats
- **Contraindications:** Wrist and/or shoulder problems

VARIATIONS & PEEL BACKS

- **Modification:** If you're less than 5'4" place moon box or roller against shoulder rests
- **Peel Backs:** *Plank, Around the World/ Up Stretch*

IMAGINE...you are a ballerina showing off your incredible leg extension with supreme control and grace.*

SUSI SAYS..."I think of this exercise as a really fancy, fun booty exercise."*

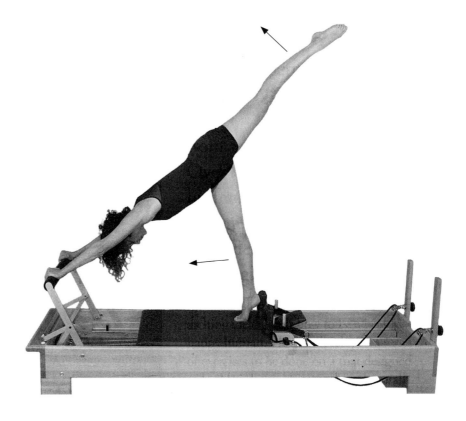

1. Starting Position—*8 repetitions each side*
Hands placed shoulder width apart on footbar, with toes on carriage and heels against shoulder rests in relevé position. Lift one foot off carriage and extend leg behind body with knee straight and foot pointed. Turn leg out at hip and raise leg as high as possible keeping both ASIS pointed to floor. Head and upper body reach through arms creating one long diagonal line from top of head to pointed toe.

2. Inhale
Push carriage out with hamstring of standing leg, maintaining the long diagonal of the body.

3. Exhale
Pull abdominals to spine stabilizing torso, pull carriage in with lower leg hip flexors and engage glute of extended leg to raise leg even higher. ROM is small and movement is performed with small pulses.

After completing 8 repetitions, switch legs by circling back leg around placing foot against shoulder rest.

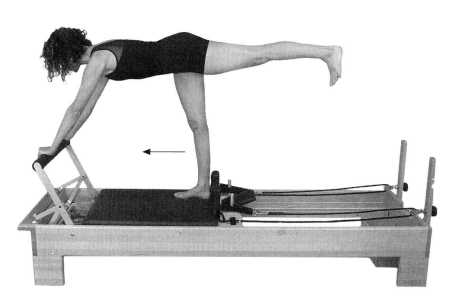

VARIATION: Arabesque in Parallel

INTERMEDIATE VARIATION:
Arabesque in Parallel
Begin in *Flat Back Elephant* and lift one leg up until it is parallel with torso. Knee cap points toward floor and foot is flexed. Use hamstring to push carriage away from home. Pull abdominals away from floor and pull standing leg forward maintaining the height of the leg and length in the torso, keeping spine in neutral. ROM is small and movement is performed with small pulses. Keep pelvis square. Do not pulse the lifted leg.

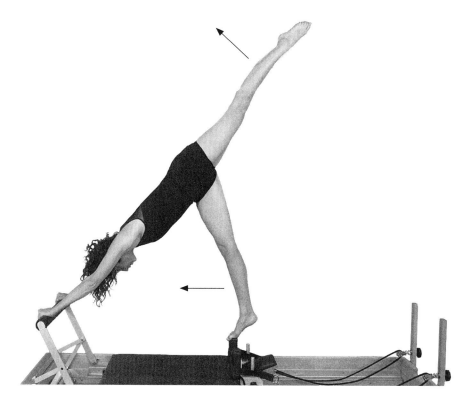

VARIATION: Arabesque on Toe on Shoulder Rest

SUPER ADVANCED VARIATION:
Arabesque on Toe on Shoulder Rest
Stand with toes on top of shoulder rest with foot in relevé. This foot position is precarious and increases the difficulty of this exercise immensely—it really challenges control and balance. It is also fun to be so high on the Reformer, but do spot your client in this position. This variation works standing quad much more than the standard position. You may want to increase resistance to accomplish this with grace.

MACHINE SET UP
- springs: 1 red & 1 blue or yellow
- bar: high
- ropes: N/A
- risers: N/A
- headrest: N/A

FUNCTIONS & TARGET MUSCLES
- Strengthens abdominals and hip flexors
- Works scapula stabilizers, hamstrings, quads, abdominals, and glutes
- Challenges client coordination
- Works knee stability

ALIGNMENT CUES & OBSTACLES
- Don't knee yourself in the face
- Breath is percussive as knee pulls toward chest—the movement is fast
- This exercise should feel like an exaggerated form of running
- Raise back leg higher to work glutes more—but keep pelvis square
- Bring leg forward with the abdominal contraction
- No rocking from side to side—weight stays even in hands
- Keep knee of standing leg aligned over 2nd & 3rd toes as it bends
- **Contraindications:** Wrist and/or shoulder problems, osteoporosis

VARIATIONS & PEEL BACKS
- **Super Advanced Variation:** *Tinkerbell:* Bend front knee into chest as carriage moves from home—as carriage pulls toward home extend bent leg up to the sky, then bend knee and arch back trying to touch toes to head

IMAGINE...*you're the winged god Mercury on the FTD logo, delivering vital messages or pretty flowers.*

ELLIE SAYS...*"This is a great advanced knee rehab—great for skiers and tennis players."*

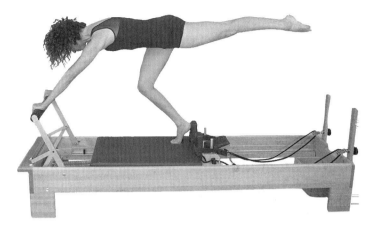

1. Starting Position—*8 to 10 repetitions*
Plank position with feet against shoulder rests with toes on carriage in relevé, hands shoulder width apart on footbar. Lift one leg behind you, bending the standing knee. Carriage remains at home.

Inhale to prepare

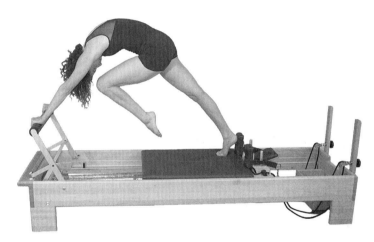

2–3. Exhale/Inhale
Pull one knee into chest as you round your back deeply imprinting abdominals to spine and send the carriage away as you straighten the standing leg—the "FTD" position. Carriage returns home as you return to Starting Position—standing leg bends and gesture leg returns to low, parallel *Arabesque*.

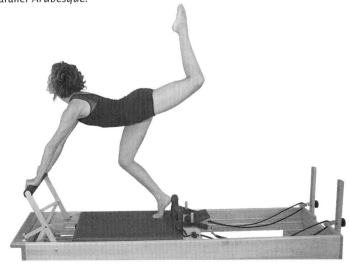

SUPER ADVANCED VARIATION: Tinkerbell

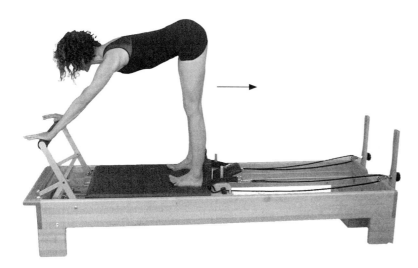

1. Starting Position—*6 to 10 repetitions*

Hands on bar, shoulder width apart or wider, fingers reaching long and wrist as straight as possible. Feet flat on carriage, heels against shoulder rests, and toes flexed off mat. Spine is straight in a flat back position.

2. Inhale

Using hamstrings push carriage out as far as possible with out changing pelvis, about 8".

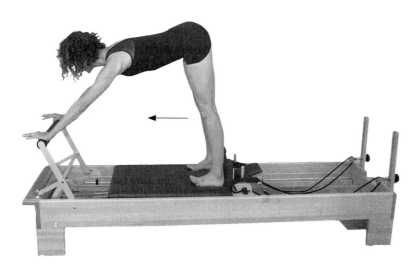

3. Exhale

Pulls abs to spine and flex at hips reaching sit bones up and back, to pull carriage toward home.

Repeat with small pulsing motions, accenting the "in" motion.

MACHINE SET UP
- spring: 1 red & 1 blue or yellow
- bar: high
- ropes: N/A
- risers: N/A
- headrest: N/A

FUNCTIONS & TARGET MUSCLES
- Strengthens hip flexors
- Works shoulder stabilizers, low abdominals, and dorsiflexors
- Stretches hamstrings
- Great for people with posterior pelvic tilt

ALIGNMENT CUES & OBSTACLES
- Keep toes lifted
- Keep belly lifted to prevent hyperextension of spine when flexing hips with psoas
- Keep arches up and lifted—do not allow ankles to roll in
- Stabilize scapulae down back keeping back and collar bone wide—this also helps keep pressure off wrists
- Avoid hyperextending or locking the elbows and knees
- **Obstacle:** Tight hamstrings—do rounded variation or raise heels into relevé position to decrease stretch on hamstrings

VARIATIONS & PEEL BACKS
- To increase hamstring stretch and challenge shoulder stability, increase bend in hips to a position similar to "downward dog"
- **Peel Back:** *Flat Back Knee Stretch*

IMAGINE...*your coccyx is a tail reaching straight out parallel to the floor, not down between your legs –or– imagine you're making a table with your spine, and someone has placed a cup of tea on your back, which you don't want to spill.*

SUSI SAYS...*"Keep the legs separate from the pelvis—flat back positions are good for those clients that like to tuck."*

ELLIE SAYS...*"It looks easy, but it is strangely not."*

ELEPHANT: ROUND BACK

MACHINE SET UP
- spring: 1 red & 1 blue or yellow
- bar: high
- ropes: N/A
- risers: N/A
- headrest: N/A

FUNCTIONS & TARGET MUSCLES
- Strengthens abdominals
- Works shoulder stabilizers, hip flexors, and dorsiflexors
- Stretches spine and hamstrings
- Great for people with anterior pelvic tilt

ALIGNMENT CUES & OBSTACLES
- Think of folding at the navel
- Keep arches up and lifted—do not allow ankles to roll in
- Stabilize scapulae down back keeping back and collar bone wide—this also helps keep pressure off wrists
- Avoid hyperextending or locking the elbows and knees

VARIATIONS & PEEL BACKS
- To increase hamstring stretch and challenge shoulder stability, increase bend in hips to a position similar to "downward dog"
- **Peel Back:** *Round Back Knee Stretch*

IMAGINE…*you imprinting your lower spine onto the ceiling.*

ELLIE SAYS…*"The lower back should be the highest point of the arch, not your tailbone. So keep your tail between your legs."*

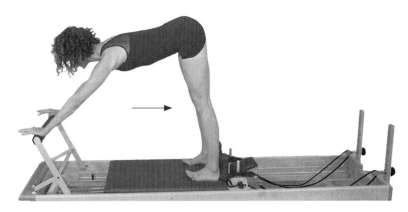

1. Starting Position—*6 to 10 repetitions*
Transition from *Flat Back Elephant* by pressing the carriage out about a foot away from home. Scoop the abdominals in and round the spine to bring carriage towards home position. Do not drop the head.

2. Inhale
Using hamstrings push carriage out as far as possible with out changing pelvis, about 8".

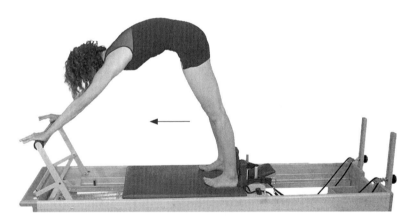

3. Exhale
Pull carriage toward home rounding the spine.

Repeat the movement of the carriage with small pulses, accenting the "in" motion.

After competing 8 repetitions, bring carriage home and continue with *Forward Bend Stretch.*

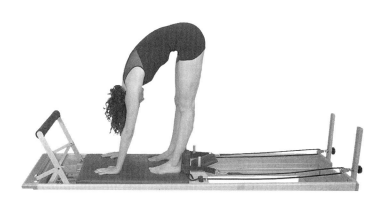

1. Starting Position—*1 repetition*
Standing with flat feet on Reformer with heels against shoulder rests. Body is folded in half.

Inhale to prepare

2. Breathing Continuously
Allow gravity to lengthen and stretch spine as you reach sit bones up to sky to increase hamstring stretch. Gently nod and/or shake head from side to side to release neck. Hold for 3 long, slow breaths.

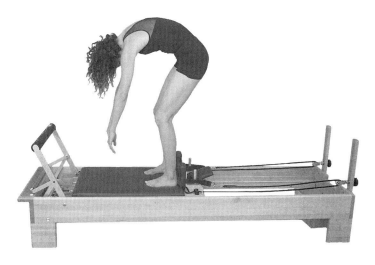

3. Exhale
Soften knees and begin to roll up sequentially through spine starting with coccyx. Allow tailbone to be heavy. End by bringing head atop spine, standing tall and relaxed.

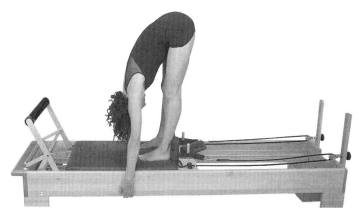

VARIATION: For the Super Flexible

MACHINE SET UP
- springs:
- bar: high
- ropes: N/A
- risers: N/A
- headrest: N/A

FUNCTIONS & TARGET MUSCLES
- Stretches hamstrings and back extensors
- Releases neck

ALIGNMENT CUES & OBSTACLES
- Keep knees soft when rolling up to standing
- Don't juice your imaginary fruit when rolling up to standing and allow scapulae sliding down your back to help you up
- Keep weight in toes—don't sink back into heels
- **Contraindications:** Unstable SI joint, disc dysfunction, osteoporosis

VARIATIONS & PEEL BACKS
- **Variation:** For the Super Flexible: To increase hamstring stretch hold onto bottom of Reformer and pull torso deeper into forward bend

IMAGINE...*your spine releasing and lengthening as gravity pulls your skull closer to the ground.*

ELLIE SAYS...*"Stand next to your client and put a hand on their back in case they feel off balance as they roll up."*

MACHINE SET UP

- springs: 1 red & 1 blue or yellow
- bar: high
- ropes: N/A
- risers: N/A
- headrest: N/A

FUNCTIONS & TARGET MUSCLES

- Strengthens triceps and lats
- Works glutes, abdominals, scapula stabilizers, and spinal extensors

ALIGNMENT CUES & OBSTACLES

- Really lift hips and push pelvis up when coming into reverse *Plank*—lead with pubic bone
- Don't allow pelvis to sink when pushing carriage out in reverse *Plank*—use your glutes
- Use lats and scapula stabilizers to keep as much weight out of wrist as possible—keep fingers long
- Feel pelvis and spine neutral as you raise and lower body in tricep press action—think: fold at hips
- Relax and stretch wrists before and after performing this exercise
- **Obstacles:** Weak triceps and lats
- **Contraindications:** Wrist issues, Carpal Tunnel Syndrome, Repetitive Stress injuries, weak and unstable shoulders

VARIATIONS & PEEL BACKS

- **Modification:** If client is less than 5"6' place a roller or moon box against shoulder rest and have client press toes into prop
- **Modification:** *Tricep Press*: In Starting Position of exercise, bend and straighten elbows, keeping carriage at home and maintaining Neutral Spine

IMAGINE...*you are drawing a right angle triangle in space with your pelvis.*

ELLIE SAYS...*"Just like the name of this exercise tells you—try to keep your back long when you're in the reverse Plank and when you're lowering or lifting body."*

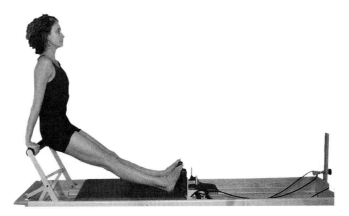

1. Starting Position—*3 reps each direction*
Seated on footbar with hands on either side of pelvis with fingers facing feet. Toes press into shoulder rests and heels pressing into carriage. Knees are straight.

Inhale wide into back and press hands into footbar to lift pelvis up

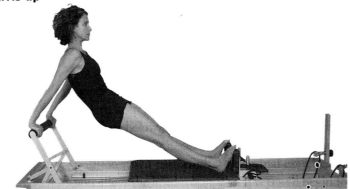

2. Exhale
Begin to push carriage away from home, bringing pubic bone toward ceiling. Glutes will be working. Move sequentially through spine from pelvis to shoulders to bring body into reverse *Plank* position, making a long diagonal from ankles to shoulders.

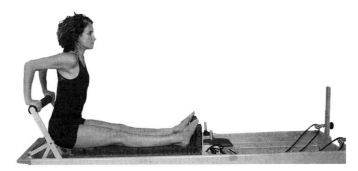

3. Inhale
Break diagonal at hip joint and lower pelvis so it hovers just above carriage. Bend elbows and bring carriage close to home. Low back is slightly rounded.

4. Exhale
Release pelvis back, bringing it into neutral (stick your booty out) and press hands into footbar, straighten elbows and lift pelvis up.

Repeat 2 more times. Then reverse the movement of the pelvis: bend elbows to lower pelvis keeping spine neutral, push carriage out and leading with the pubic bone lift and snake torso into reverse *Plank*, then bring carriage home maintaining reverse *Plank* as long as possible, return to Starting Position by releasing pelvis into neutral.

stomach massage series

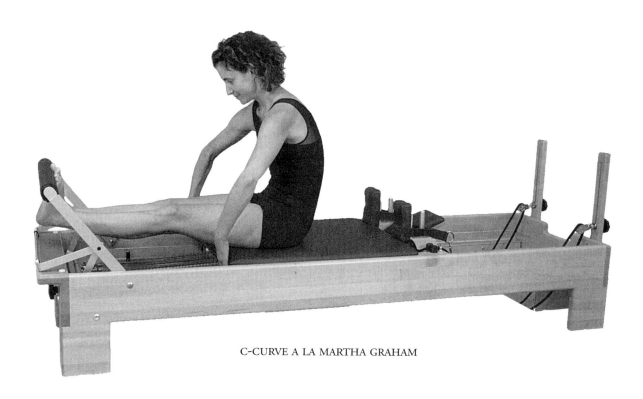

C-CURVE A LA MARTHA GRAHAM

MARTHA GRAHAM SAID,
"WHETHER YOU LAUGH OR CRY, YOUR CENTER IS INVOLVED."

The Stomach Massage Series is similar to the floor exercises of modern dance pioneer Martha Graham. She revolutionized the modern dance world by introducing the "contraction"—basically spinal flexion. In Pilates we call it the C-Curve. Her intense floor work emphasized lifting the spine off the pelvis using the deep postural muscles and initiating movement from the center of the body (abdominal muscles).

This series is performed seated on a sticky pad placed one hand's distance from the front edge of the carriage. Toes are on the low bar with feet in Pilates "V"—hips and knees starting in deep flexion. People with tight hamstrings will hate this exercise. A *Psoas Stretch* after this series is a welcome relief.

BEGINNING
Round Back
Flat Back

INTERMEDIATE
Reaching
Bouquet

ROUND BACK

MACHINE SET UP
- springs: 2 red & 1 blue or yellow
- bar: low
- ropes: N/A
- risers: N/A
- headrest: N/A

FUNCTIONS & TARGET MUSCLES
- Strengthens abdominals while stretching spinal extensors
- Works spine in deep flexion and reinforces concept of C-Curve
- Works hip flexors, external hip rotators, adductors and quads
- Stretches and strengthens plantar flexors and hamstrings
- Enables client to observe knee and ankle alignment through a large Range of Motion

ALIGNMENT CUES & OBSTACLES
- Knees should follow alignment of the feet— don't let knees fall open and don't over rotate at the ankles
- Use abdominals to round spine into deep C-Curve keeping head over pelvis
- Keep the feeling of length
- Keep head following the line of the spine
- Keep heels connected during entire exercise
- Don't "hold on for dear life" with hands
- Use abdominals to resist the springs as the carriage returns to home
- It's called *Stomach Massage* because you are thinking of massaging your organs with your deep abdominals
- **Obstacles:** Tight hamstrings, tight/weak low back
- **Contraindications:** disc dysfunction, osteoporosis

VARIATIONS & PEEL BACKS
- **Modification:** If client is tight, move sticky pad and Starting Position farther away from the edge of the carriage
- **Peel Backs:** *C-Curve Pulse* on the Cadillac and *Spine Stretch Forward* on the Mat are excellent peel backs for this exercise, as is any exercise that focuses on spinal flexion

IMAGINE...*a cannon ball is shot at your abdomen to initiate the movement, and you must return the cannon ball home safely by hugging it with your abs.*

ELLIE SAYS...*"I call this Martha Graham meets the Reformer. Do it for Martha. Feel your abs for Martha!"*

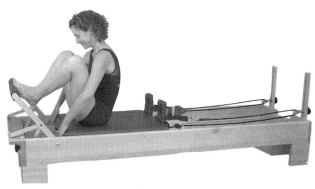

1. Starting Position—*6 repetitions*
Sitting on sit bones, toes on bar with feet in Pilates "V", hips externally rotated and deeply flexed with knees bent. Entire spine is in C-Curve. Hands placed outside of legs, holding onto front edge of carriage.

Inhale to prepare

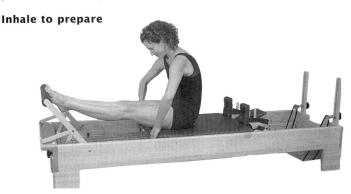

2. Exhale
Pull abdominals to spine and deepen the sense of C-Curve as you push away from bar, straightening legs, keeping heels high. Don't roll behind sit bones.

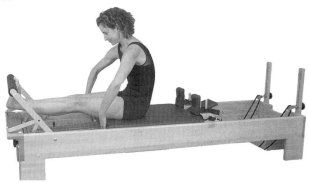

3. Inhale
Lower heels under bar without bending knees.

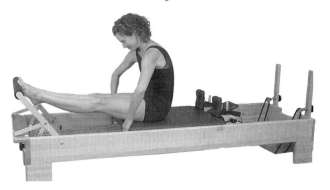

4–5. Exhale/Inhale
Exhale as you raise heels and increase abdominal contraction, then inhale bending knees to control carriage home.

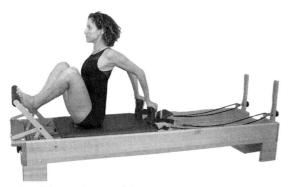

1. Starting Position—*6 repetitions*

Toes on bar with feet in Pilates "V", hips externally rotated and deeply flexed with knees deeply bent. Spine straight, shoulders rotated open, hands on shoulder rests with fingers away from body. The chest is very open with the upper back in slight extension. Keep elbows bent and pointed back.

Inhale to prepare by lifting torso out of hips

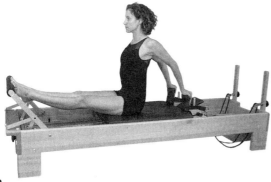

2. Exhale

Pull abdominals to spine increasing sense of torso length, push away from bar, straightening legs and keeping heels high.

3. Inhale

Lower heels under bar without bending knees.

4–5. Exhale/Inhale

Exhale as you raise heels and increase abdominal engagement. Inhale, then bend knees to bring the carriage home.

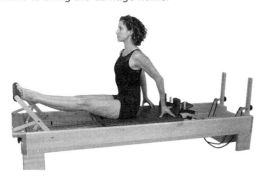

VARIATION: Spider Fingers

After 2 repetitions change to "*Spider Fingers*" (fingertips on carriage with palms pulled up away from carriage, fingertips point away from body), hands a little wider than shoulder rests, which provide less support than the above position.

MODIFICATION: PhysioBall

MACHINE SET UP
- springs: 2 red
- bar: low
- rope: N/A
- risers: N/A
- headrest: N/A

FUNCTIONS & TARGET MUSCLES
- Strengthens spinal extensors, abdominals in a lengthened position, and psoas which is working to maintain seated position
- Opens chest and works shoulder girdle stabilizers
- Works hip flexors, external hip rotators, adductors, and quads
- Stretches and strengthens plantar flexors and hamstrings
- Enables client to observe knee and ankle alignment through a large Range of Motion

ALIGNMENT CUES & OBSTACLES
- Keep shoulders down and weight off of fingers by lifting the torso with abdominals and back
- Keep heels connected for entire exercise
- Pull inner thighs together as knees straighten
- Exaggerate the straightness of the upper back with a bit of upper back extension (similar to *Flat Back* in *Roll Down* series on Cadillac and Springboard)
- This is a great exercise for pregnant clients—in 3rd trimester widen feet to 2nd position (heels at the corners of the bar)
- Don't lean on arms—keep elbows soft and pointing back
- Each inhale is a chance for torso to lengthen away from pelvis
- **Obstacles:** Tight hamstrings, weak low back, weak psoas

VARIATIONS & PEEL BACKS
- **Modification:** Put a small PhysioBall between clients back and shoulder rest for support if needed
- **Modification:** Place client farther than a hand's distance from carriage edge if hips are inflexible and/or low back is really weak

IMAGINE...*you have a stick up your butt.*

SUSI SAYS...*"If they don't like this exercise, it probably means they NEED to do it."*

MACHINE SET UP
- springs: 2 red
- bar: low
- rope: N/A
- risers: N/A
- headrest: N/A

FUNCTIONS & TARGET MUSCLES
- Strengthens spinal extensor muscles and abdominals in a lengthened position
- Strengthens psoas
- Works shoulder girdle stabilizers
- Works hip flexors, external hip rotators, adductors and quads
- Stretches and strengthens plantar flexors and hamstrings
- Enables client to observe knee and ankle alignment through a large Range of Motion

ALIGNMENT CUES & OBSTACLES
- On first few repetitions, hold client's hands and pull them forward for a deep stretch
- Keep shoulders down, back straight and energy through the spine
- **Obstacles:** Tight hamstrings, tight lats, and weak psoas
- **Contraindications:** Neck problems, tight upper traps, disc dysfunction, osteoporosis

VARIATIONS & PEEL BACKS
- If tight hamstrings prevent leaning forward, keep torso upright with arms straight overhead
- **Peel Backs:** *Salute, Round Back Stomach Massage*

IMAGINE...*your body is a ray (remember geometry) and you have energy arrows shooting out your feet, spine, and hands.*

ELLIE SAYS...*"You are reversing your spinal curves here...lumbar spine curves into flexion, thoracic spine extends."*

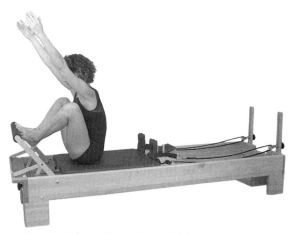

1. Starting Position—*6 to 8 repetitions*
Toes on bar with feet in Pilates "V", hips externally rotated and deeply flexed, with knees deeply bent. Spine pitches forward so body is at approximately a 60° angle. Arms reach overhead continuing the line of the spine in a wide "V". Widen arms if necessary to keep shoulders down and away from ears.

Inhale to prepare and lengthen spine away from pelvis

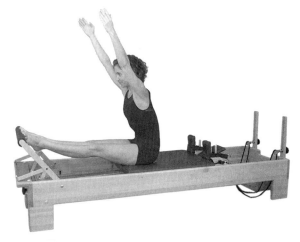

2. Exhale
Keeping heels high, straighten knees and push bar away, feeling a deep C-Curve in lumbar spine and pulling inner thighs together. Note that you *don't* lower heels on this exercise.

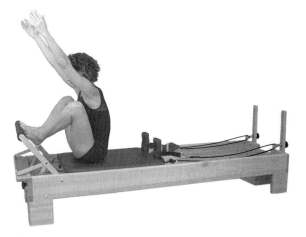

3. Inhale
Control carriage home and repeat.

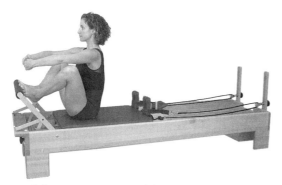

1. Starting Position—*6 to 8 repetitions*
Toes on bar with feet in Pilates "V", hips externally rotated and deeply flexed with knees deeply bent. Spine straight with arms in front of body, hands just below sternum, elbows rounded (middle fifth ballet arms) as if you are holding a huge *Bouquet* of flowers.

Inhale and lift spine away from pelvis

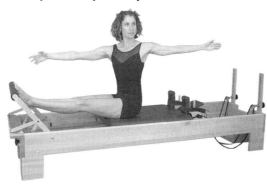

2. Exhale
Straighten legs, keep heels high and together while twisting rib cage, open arms to the sides (second position ballet arms). Note that you *don't* lower heels on this exercise.

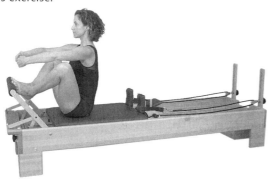

3. Inhale
Return carriage to home while untwisting and lengthening spine, bring arms back to Starting Position.

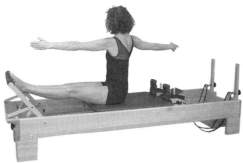

4. Exhale
Repeat, twisting to other side.

MACHINE SET UP
- springs: 2 red
- bar: low
- rope: N/A
- risers: N/A
- headrest: N/A

FUNCTIONS & TARGET MUSCLES
- Strengthens spinal muscles, and abdominals in a lengthened position
- Works internal and external obliques as well as quadratus lumborum
- Works hip flexors, external hip rotators, adductors, and quads
- Stretches and strengthens plantar flexors and hamstrings
- Teaches twisting through ribcage/thoracic spine while stabilizing pelvis

ALIGNMENT CUES & OBSTACLES
- Hold client's hand as they rotate and reach away from you
- Feel the spine lengthen to create the twist
- Keep pelvis square as ribs rotate
- **Obstacles:** Tight hamstrings, hips, obliques, QL, and/or weak lumbar spine, psoas
- **Contraindications:** Lumbar disc problems, osteoporosis

VARIATIONS & PEEL BACKS
- You can begin the exercise with the arms overhead (in high 5th position), and open them to side as you push out to straighten leg—this helps to emphasize the lift in the spine
- **Variation: Stretches:** Finish the series and place hands on footbar. Straighten knees, stretching out back muscles, hamstrings and calves. Bend one knee to increase the stretch on the opposite leg. Really reach through the heels to increase the stretch
- **Peel Backs:** *Flat Back Stomach Massage, Old Man at the Gym, Twist with Stick*

IMAGINE...you're holding a Bouquet of flowers and twisting to offer a bloom to your beloved behind you.

ELLIE SAYS...*"Spot your clients—they love it when you hold their hand!"*

PSOAS STRETCH

MACHINE SET UP
- springs: 1 red or 1 red & 1 yellow
- bar: high
- ropes: N/A
- risers: N/A
- headrest: N/A

FUNCTIONS & TARGET MUSCLES
- Stretches hip flexors
- Peel back for *Splits Series*

ALIGNMENT CUES & OBSTACLES
- Keep pelvis square to the front
- Maintain one long line from knee to the top of head while pulling carriage home—do not break at the hip
- Squeeze glutes and tuck pelvis under to increase stretch
- Think: runner's lunge stretch, with Reformer adding resistance
- Do not bend front knee past 90° or allow standing ankle to roll in or out

VARIATIONS & PEEL BACKS
- With carriage home, circle arm to the outside. Keep pelvis square as torso twists with arm. Hold position/twist when arm is parallel to floor
- **Variation:** *Dural Stretch*: On last repetition with the carriage in home position, keep spine long and slowly roll down from the top of head until you feel a deep *Psoas Stretch* in your back. By rounding the cervical and thoracic spine you are creating tension in the whole spine, thus causing the dura mater (covering of the spinal cord) to stretch. The psoas attaches to the lumbar spine so you should feel the stretch at the lumbar attachments

IMAGINE...*your ASIS are headlights and keep them facing forward.*

ELLIE SAYS...*"If a client is feeling pressure in the knee, chances are high they're not using their abdominals to lift and support the torso up and out of the knee."*

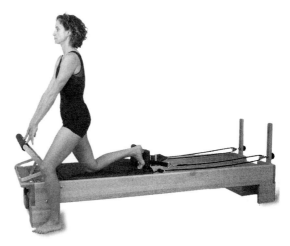

1. Starting Position
Place hands on footbar. Standing to the side of Reformer with one foot even with front edge, bend knee directly over ankle. Place the other foot against shoulder rest with the knee bent and resting on the carriage.

2. Breathing continuously
Press foot into shoulder rest and move carriage away from home, keeping front knee bent over the ankle (the angle should never be lower than 90°). Hold back leg in extension for a few rounds of breath, increasing low abdominal engagement and squeezing glutes on each exhale to maximize the stretch. Keep torso up and lifted to keep weight out of back knee.

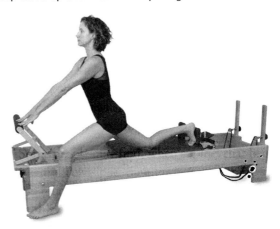

3. Exhale
Tuck pelvis under using glutes and slowly draw carriage home, bringing torso forward and up, returning to Starting Position. Do not round upper back or flex the hip.

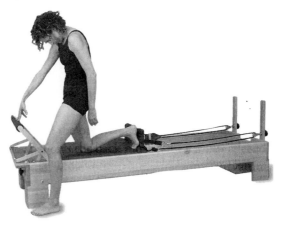

VARIATION: Dural Stretch

knee stretch series

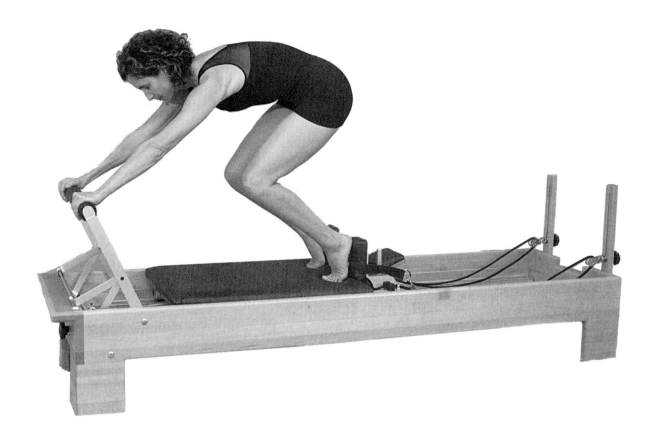

Knee Stretch Series stretches and strengthens the quads. Be careful of your knees: if you feel compression, skip the *Round Back/Flat Back* variations and just do the more advanced *Knees Off* variation. Remember: use low bar (except for *Scooter*). If you are smaller than 5'4", you can use high bar or put a roller at the shoulder rests.

Choose either classic *Knee Stretches* or *Reverse Knee Stretches*. Don't do both in an hour workout!

KNEE STRETCHES
Scooter
Flat Back Knee Stretch
Round Back Stretch
Knees Off

SCOOTER: FLAT BACK/ROUND BACK *knee stretch series*

MACHINE SET UP
- springs: 1 red or 1 red & 1 yellow
- bar: high
- ropes: N/A
- risers: N/A
- headrest: N/A

FUNCTIONS & TARGET MUSCLES
- Strengthens glute max, hamstrings, and quads
- Stretches hip flexors
- Great for knee rehabilitation

ALIGNMENT CUES & OBSTACLES
- Focus on femur moving into extension while pelvis and lumbar spine remain neutral and stable
- Press through heel and really focus on the glute max firing

VARIATIONS & PEEL BACKS
- **Variation:** *Turn Out:* Externally rotate both hips, back toes make contact with shoulder rest, heel is high, and knee points to the side, rather than down. Standing leg makes half of the Pilates "V". Maintain pelvic stability—rotation happens at the hip, not lumbar spine

IMAGINE...*your ASIS are headlights shining forward.*

SUSI SAYS...*"This is such a great exercise for all those 'tuckers' out there. Since the pelvis is neutral rather than retroverted the lumbar erectors have to work to maintain Neutral Spine."*

ELLIE SAYS...*"This is a kinder, gentler, one-legged Knee Stretch. Perfect for those who can't kneel or for injured and sensitive knees."*

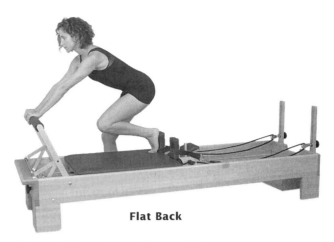

Flat Back

1. Starting Position—*10 to 15 repetitions*
In lunge position on Reformer like *Psoas Stretch* except knee is lifted off carriage, and standing leg is farther back, about 2' from the front of Reformer.

Inhale and lengthen spine to prepare

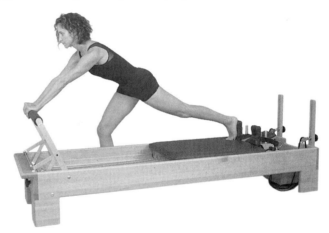

2-3. Exhale/Inhale
Exale as you pull abdominals to spine and push carriage out as far as possible, keeping pelvis square and spine neutral. Really focus on glute contracting and moving from the femur, not from the low back. Inhale as you release leg and return to Starting Position.

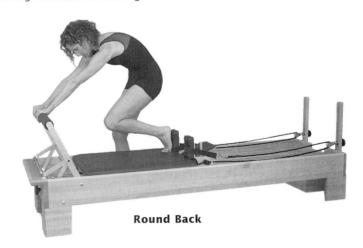

Round Back

For *Round Back* version: Place both hands on footbar, rounding spine. Keeping back knee lifted, straighten back leg pushing carriage away from home. Push heel into shoulder rest to focus work on hamstrings and glutes. Use heavier springs for this version.

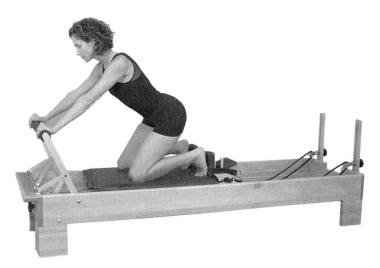

1. Starting Position—*6 to 10 repetitions*
Kneel on carriage with feet against shoulder rests with toes forward and hands on footbar, shoulder width apart. Spine is in neutral with abdominals pulling away from floor. Sit bones reach up and back.

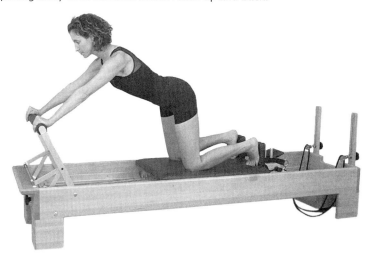

2. Inhale
Push carriage away from home using legs and maintaining Neutral Spine.

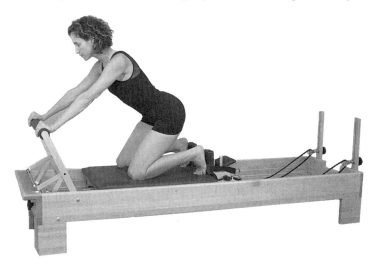

3. Exhale
Engage abdominals to spine and pull femurs toward hands, without flexing or arching the lumbar spine, accenting the "in" movement, bringing the carriage almost all the way home, returning to Starting Position.

MACHINE SET UP
- springs: 1 red & 1 blue or yellow
- bar: low
- ropes: N/A
- risers: N/A
- headrest: N/A

FUNCTIONS & TARGET MUSCLES
- Strengthens spinal extensors, psoas and abs
- Works scapula stabilizers, quads, low abdominals
- Peel back for *Plank Series*
- Teaches Neutral Spine
- Great for "tuckers"

ALIGNMENT CUES & OBSTACLES
- Keep spine neutral as femurs move out and in
- Stick your booty out—think: sit bones toward heels, not toward knees
- Keep upper body stable and relaxed—don't crunch back of neck
- Even though the spine is neutral, pull abdominals up to spine away from floor— don't hyperextend lumbar spine
- **Contraindications:** Knee injuries

IMAGINE...*your tail is in the air, pointing straight like a hunting dog.*

SUSI SAYS...*"This is a great peel back for the Elephant and or any exercise which requires clients to bear weight in their hands."*

MACHINE SET UP
- springs: 1 red & 1 blue or yellow
- bar: low
- ropes: N/A
- risers: N/A
- headrest: N/A

FUNCTIONS & TARGET MUSCLES
- Works scapula stabilizers, quads, and low abdominals
- Peel back for *Plank Series*
- Stretches spinal extensors and quads

ALIGNMENT CUES & OBSTACLES
- Maintain full spine C-Curve—do not collapse chin into chest
- Use abdominals to maintain spinal flexion—don't lose curve when legs go out
- Do not hyperextend elbows—keep elbow creases facing each other
- **Contraindications:** Knee injuries, arthritis or sensitivity, disc dysfunction, osteoporosis

IMAGINE...*you are a dog with your tail between your legs.*

ELLIE SAYS...*"This is the easiest way to find the C-Curve."*

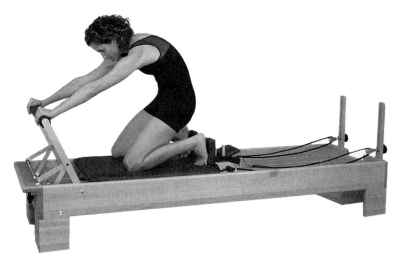

1. Starting Position—*6 to 10 repetitions*
Kneel on carriage with feet against shoulder rests, toes forward, hands on footbar shoulder width apart. Entire spine is rounded into a full C-Curve. You should be almost sitting on your heels, but feel your spine "inflated" up off your legs.

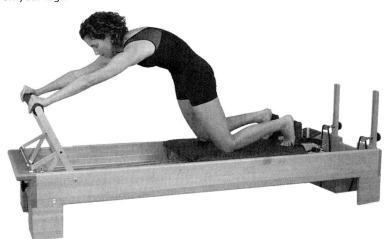

2. Inhale
Maintain spinal curve and push carriage away from home using hamstrings.

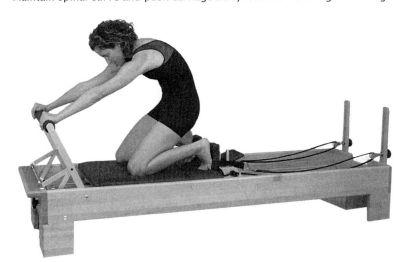

3. Exhale
Pull abdominals to spine and accent the "in" movement, deepening spinal flexion, returning to Starting Position, without coming all the way home.

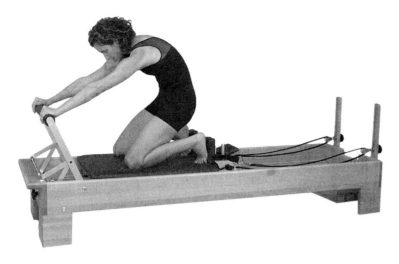

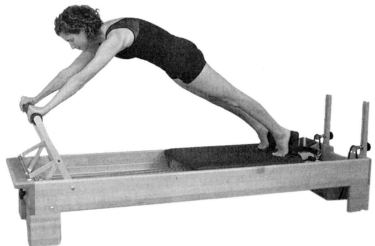

1. Starting Position—*10 to 20 repetitions*
Transition from *Round Back Knee Stretches*: press carriage all the way out, and lift knees off carriage, pressing out to the *Plank* in one fell swoop.

Inhale to prepare

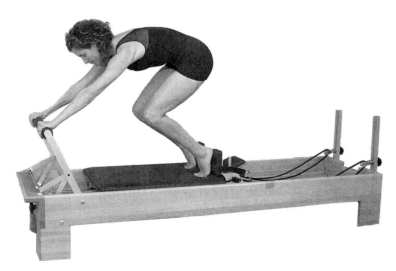

2. Exhale
Pull carriage home maintaining lumbar flexion and bringing knees toward chest. Really scoop out low abdominals.

MACHINE SET UP
- springs: 1 red & 1 blue
- bar: low
- ropes: N/A
- risers: N/A
- headrest: N/A

FUNCTIONS & TARGET MUSCLES
- Strengthens spinal extensors and hip flexors
- Works scapula stabilizers, quads, and low abdominals
- Great for skiers!

ALIGNMENT CUES & OBSTACLES
- Isolate movement at hip and knee joint— keep upper body stable
- Push heels into shoulder rests when straightening legs to engage hamstrings and glutes
- Keep scapulae stable and jaw relaxed
- Do not lock elbows
- Keep knees as close to carriage as possible—lower knees equals more work
- The lower spine is rounding but the upper spine is straight
- **Contraindications:** Wrist and/or shoulder injuries, patellar tracking injuries, osteoporosis

VARIATIONS & PEEL BACKS
- **Modifications:** Work with pelvis high in an *Elephant* position (requires less upper body strength)
- **Peel Backs:** *Plank, Knee Stretches, Elephant*

IMAGINE...*your knees are in tracks—sliding back and forth in two lines.*

ELLIE SAYS...*"In New York, they once made me do as many repetitions as my age...oy vey!"*

reverse knee stretch series

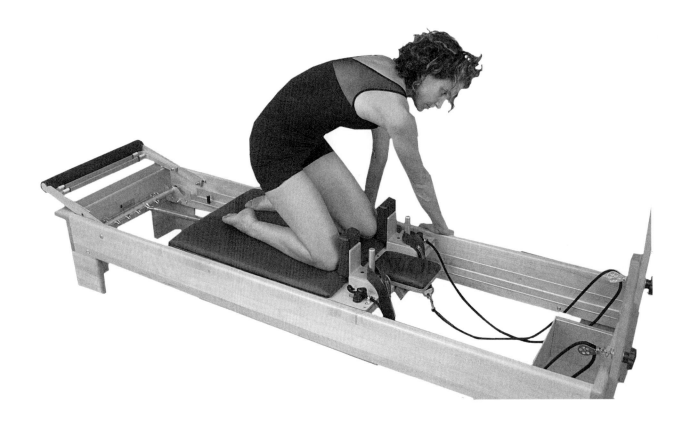

Reverse Knee Stretches are a great alternative to the classical *Knee Stretches* because they are much less loaded on the knees. The name of this series is a bit misleading since these exercises actually strengthen the abdominals and hip flexors more than they stretch the knee. They are the least loaded spinal flexion exercises in the Reformer repertoire, so they're great for pregnant women and people with spinal injuries. The *Oblique* variation is great for scoliosis and pelvic imbalances.

Choose either classic *Knee Stretches* or *Reverse Knee Stretches*. Don't do both in an hour workout!

REVERSE KNEE STRETCHES
Round Back
Flat Back
Obliques

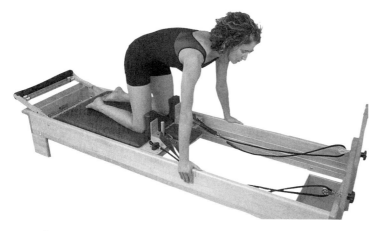

1. Starting Position—*6 to 8 repetitions*

On all fours, facing back of Reformer, with knees against shoulder rests and hands holding frame, fingertips and thumbs on outside of frame. Shoulders are directly above hands and hips are directly above knees. Hollow upper back a bit to encourage serratus anterior to engage.

Inhale to prepare

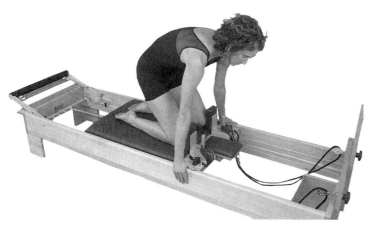

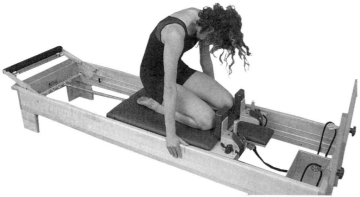

2. Exhale

Start the motion like a cat pulling its tail between its legs, initiate a *Coccyx Curl* and pull abdominals deeply toward spine, rounding back sequentially from tail to head to pull knees toward hands. The carriage moves because the spine rounds, not because the arms pull. Keep pulling until you are sitting on your heels.

3. Inhale

Control carriage back to home, unfurling spine from top to tail, returning to Starting Position.

MACHINE SET UP
- springs: 1 yellow or 1 blue
- bar: N/A
- ropes: N/A
- risers: N/A
- headrest: N/A

FUNCTIONS & TARGET MUSCLES
- Strengthens abdominals
- Works shoulder stabilizers
- Stretches spinal extensors

ALIGNMENT CUES & OBSTACLES
- Do not pull with arms—that's cheating
- Move sequentially through spine without losing control at end of ROM in both directions
- Keep shoulders stable and away from ears

VARIATIONS & PEEL BACKS
- **Variation:** Pulses: start in your deep C-Curve, sitting on your heels. Come back one third the distance, and pulse back into the C-Curve, scooping your abdominals deeply on each pulse. Repeat 8 times
- **Peel Back:** *Hunting Cat* on the Mat
- **Contraindications:** Knee injuries

IMAGINE...*you're pulling your tail between your legs to initiate the movement.*

ELLIE SAYS...*"This is a great abdominal exercise for pregnant clients or clients with tailbone injuries or herniated disks. Why? 'Cuz it's not-so-loaded flexion."*

Flat Back (Beginning/Intermediate)
Maintain Neutral Spine and upper body stability as the legs pull towards hands on an exhale, femur flexes but pelvis remains still. ROM is small. To focus the action of hip flexion on the psoas, place knees directly under hips and place a small ball between inner thighs.
Single Leg Flat Back (Advanced) (not shown) Extend one leg straight back in parallel, keeping hips square, and pull the carriage in with other leg.

Flat Back 1

Flat Back 2

Obliques (Beginning/Intermediate)
Place hands on one side of frame with fingertips and thumbs pointed toward outside of frame. Place hands under shoulders, approximately 8" apart, and close to carriage. Spine bends and twists toward hands. Hollow upper back a bit to encourage serratus anterior to engage but keep back of neck long. On exhale scoop abdominals and pull tailbone straight under you as you round your lumbar spine, moving carriage away from home. Increase spinal rotation toward hands, stretching opposite side of back. This exercise feels like paddling a canoe with your abdominals. Remember—great for scoliosis!

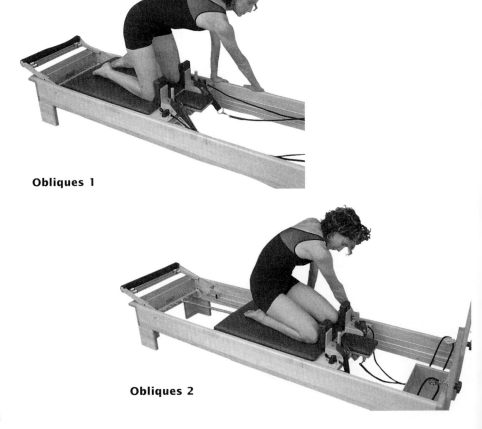

Obliques 1

Obliques 2

kneeling series

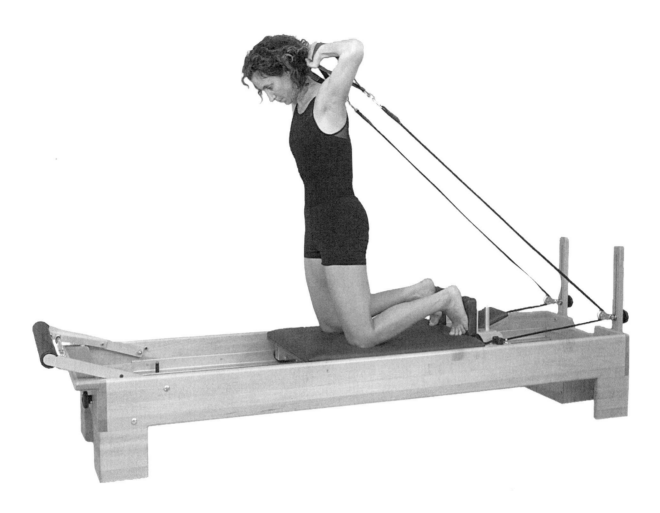

The Kneeling Series really reveals a client's postural tendencies because kneeling is a unstable position. The Pilates kneeling exercises are always done with the Powerhouse engaged; femurs pressing forward in the hip sockets (using hamstrings and glutes), abdominals scooped in, and the torso slightly pitched forward to enhance the core challenge.

Don't do more than 4 kneeling exercises in an hour workout. Too much kneeling can injure the knee. Be careful with knee issues! You can do most of these exercises sitting cross-legged on the carriage or straddling the long box. You can also put more padding (like a pillow) under the sensitive client's knees. Some of these exercises are much harder than they look (*Arm Circles, Salute*). Scary!

INTERMEDIATE	**ADVANCED**	**SUPER ADVANCED**
Chest Expansion	*Arm Circles*	*Kneeling Backbend*
La Croix	*Salute*	
Rotator		

CHEST EXPANSION

MACHINE SET UP
- springs: 1 red or 1 blue
- bar: N/A
- ropes: standard length
- risers: down
- headrest: N/A

FUNCTIONS & TARGET MUSCLES
- Strengthens lats, triceps, and rotator cuff
- Works hamstrings, glutes, and abdominals
- Challenges balance

ALIGNMENT CUES & OBSTACLES
- Do not crease at hips—really push femurs forward from the hamstrings to maintain one long line from knees to top of the head
- When kneeling, it is more difficult to maintain stability when returning to Starting Position—spot your client
- Focus on spine lengthening while moving arms—feel that invisible thread
- Keep neck relaxed and long—no forward head
- Place a rolled up pad under client's knees if kneeling causes any pain in patella—if that doesn't help, do the seated version
- **Obstacles:** Weak glutes, and poor sense of balance
- **Contraindications:** Some knee injuries (kneeling compresses the joint)

VARIATIONS & PEEL BACKS
- **Modification:** *Chest Expansion* kneeling with knees against shoulder rests
- **Peel Back:** *Chest Expansion* seated on Long Box

ELLIE SAYS... *"Now this is really the 'perfect alignment' exercise."*

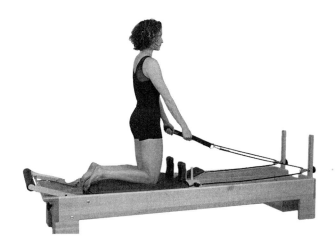

1. Starting Position—*4 repetitions*
Kneeling with feet flexed and toes holding the front edge of the carriage. Hold the folded loops, pinkies facing back. Pitch forward slightly to engage hamstrings and glutes.

Inhale and lengthen spine

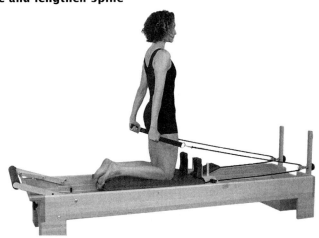

2. Exhale
Stabilize torso with abdominals, and pull arms back until even with sides (or a little further). Feel shoulders "smile" open. Pull the head of the humerus back in the shoulder socket.

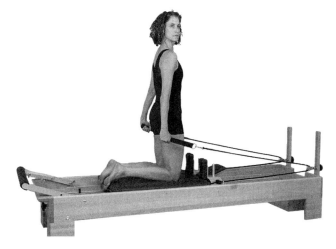

3. Breathing Continuously
Look slowly from side to side, then look straight. Do not lean back or bend at hips while returning arms to Starting Position.

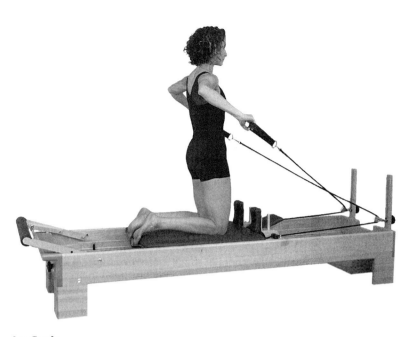

La Croix

See Seated Long Box pages 76 and 77 for alignment details.

La Croix

Kneeling with feet flexed and toes holding the front edge of the carriage. Ropes crossed, hands holding loops with elbows bent and opened to the sides, making a diamond shape with arms. Pitch forward slightly to engage hamstrings and glutes. Pull abdominals to spine, stabilizing the rib cage, and gently squeeze scapulae together, maintaining diamond shape of arms. Return to Starting Position, relaxing rhomboids, allowing scapulae to glide apart.

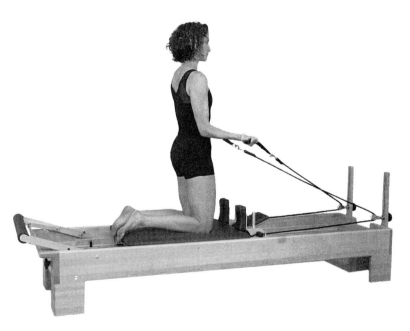

Rotator

Rotator

Kneeling with feet flexed and toes holding the front edge of the carriage. Ropes crossed, loops held with palms up and loop ends next to thumbs—the "hitch-hiker hold." Elbows bent to 90° and glued to sides. Pitch forward slightly to engage hamstrings and glutes. Stabilize rib cage by pulling abdominals toward spine. Roll humerus back, allowing forearms to rotate to sides, keeping forearms parallel to floor. Elbows do not move away from sides. Control arms back slowly to Starting Position.

MACHINE SET UP
- springs: 1 red or 1 blue
- bar: N/A
- ropes: standard length
- risers: down
- headrest: N/A

FUNCTIONS & TARGET MUSCLES
- Strengthens deltoids and scapula stabilizers
- Works abdominals, glutes and hamstrings
- Challenges balance and control

ALIGNMENT CUES & OBSTACLES
- Really pitch forward as far as you can to work back of legs and to maximize the challenge of this exercise—feel the abdominals supporting the torso
- Warm up with 2–3 *Queen* arm reaches in this position before making full *Circles*
- Keep arms in front of torso when opening arms and lowering them to sides
- Maintain even pressure of hands in loops through out the *Arm Circle*—use resistance to aid stabilization
- Move smoothly and with control—quick, jerking motions destabilize torso
- **Contraindications:** Some knee injuries (kneeling compresses the joint)

VARIATIONS & PEEL BACKS
- **Peel Backs:** *Queen, Kneeling Chest Expansion, Modified Front Rowing, Offering*

IMAGINE…*you're being supported by a strong wind blowing against the front of your body—lean in to the wind.*

ELLIE SAYS…*"Press your heels like 'brakes' into shoulder rests to help stabilize."*

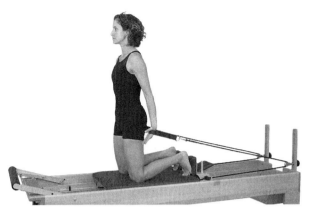

1. Starting Position—*3 repetitions in each direction*
Kneel facing front footbar with feet on shoulder rests and toes tucked forward. Press heels into shoulder rests to engage hamstrings and glutes. Pitch forward slightly. Arms are by sides with hands through loops (or handles), palms facing up and wrists are long.

Inhale to prepare

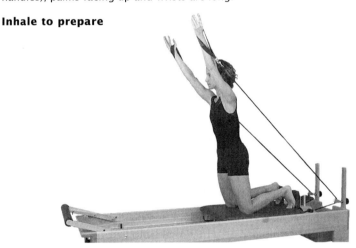

2. Exhale
Pull abdominals to spine, engage glutes and hamstrings, stabilize scapulae, and press arms forward and overhead (*Queen* reach). Keep palms facing up and feel scoop coming from scapulae.

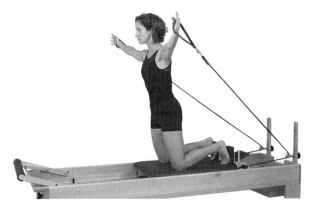

3. Exhale
Open arms out to sides with palms facing front and lower hands to sides returning to Starting Position. Maintain forward pitch of body while lowering the arms.

Repeat twice more, and then reverse direction of *Arm Circles*.

Note: When lowering arms in front of the body on reverse *Arm Circles*, palms should face up to facilitate open chest and stable scapulae.

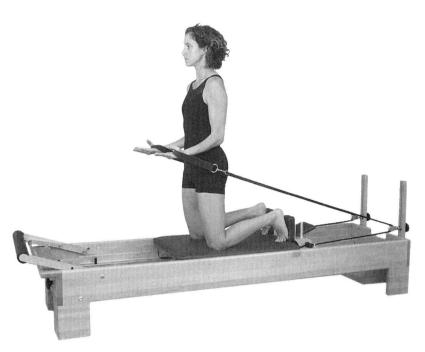

MODIFICATION: Offering
(Intermediate) Begin with elbows by
sides and forearms parallel to floor.
Reach arms forward like you are
Offering a tray of margaritas to a
party guest. Be sure not to lean back
as you reach forward. Return arms to
Starting Position.

MODIFICATION: Offering 1

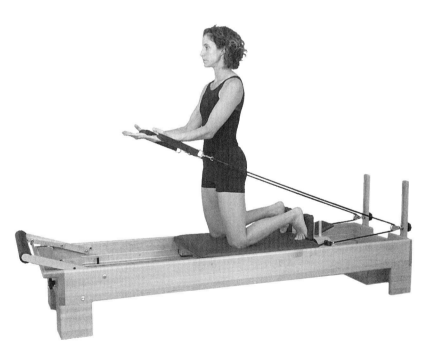

MODIFICATION: Offering 2

MACHINE SET UP

- springs: 1 red or 1 blue
- bar: N/A
- ropes: standard length
- risers: down
- headrest: N/A

FUNCTIONS & TARGET MUSCLES

- Strengthens triceps and deltoids
- Works abdominals, glutes, hamstrings, and mid traps
- Challenges balance and control

ALIGNMENT CUES & OBSTACLES

- Carriage will not be in home position at start of exercise
- Move smoothly and with control—quick, jerking motions destabilize torso
- This is a precarious position, so spot your client
- Focus on the mid traps keeping scapulae stable
- Maintain pressure of arms in straps to stabilize when bending elbows
- To decrease pressure on patellae, kneel upright, not pitched forward
- **Obstacles:** Tight lats, weak glutes, fear of falling
- **Contraindications:** Some knee injuries (kneeling compresses the joint)

VARIATIONS & PEEL BACKS

- **Variation:** *Shave the Head:* Drop head forward bringing hands behind head and *Salute* the Pilates goddess from this position (like you're shaving off the back of your head)
- **Peel Backs:** *Salute* seated on the Long Box, Kneeling Chest Expansion

IMAGINE...*you are a figurine carved into the prow of a ship and the entire ship supports you as you lean forward.*

ELLIE SAYS...*"Scary!"*

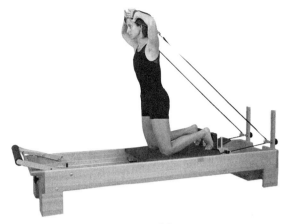

1. Starting Position—*4 repetitions*

Kneel facing footbar, with feet against shoulder rests and toes tucked forward. Press heels into shoulder rests to engage hamstrings and glutes, and lean forward as far as you can. With hands in loops, *Salute* forehead with elbows bent and index fingers touching eyebrows. Palms face out.

Inhale to prepare

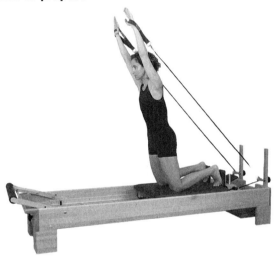

2–3. Exhale/Inhale

Exhale as you pull abdominals to spine, push heels into shoulder rests to engage glutes and hamstrings, and stabilize scapulae while straightening elbows, keeping arms in line with body. Inhale to bend elbows and bring hands back to forehead while maintaining pitch of the body.

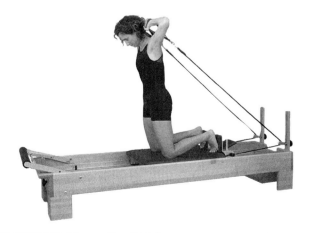

VARIATION: Shave the Head

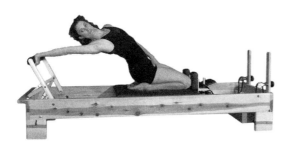

1. Starting Position—*once with 5 push ups*
Sit on heels with knees against shoulder rests. Reach one arm back to grab under the footbar, palm facing up. Push carriage out as far as possible while still sitting on heels.

Inhale to prepare

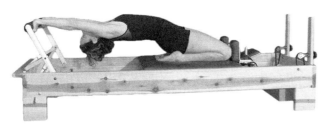

2. Exhale
Keeping pelvis tucked under, lay out your torso, looking back to the footbar, and grab under the footbar with other hand.

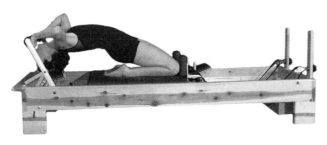

3. Breathing Continuously
Bend elbows to sides, allowing head to come under footbar as you maintain your tucked pelvis by scooping the belly in and engaging your glutes. Do 5 push ups by bending and extending your elbows.

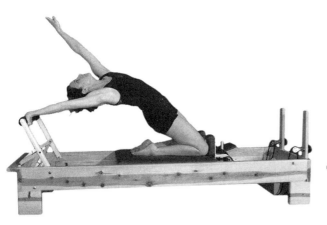

4. Exhale
To finish, after your fifth push up, release one arm up to the sky as you lift torso, allowing carriage to come home.

MACHINE SET UP
- springs: 2 red or 1 red & 1 blue
- bar: high
- ropes: N/A
- risers: N/A
- headrest: N/A

FUNCTIONS & TARGET MUSCLES
- Stretches the abdominals, hip flexors, chest, lats, and pecs
- Strengthens the glutes, lower back, shoulders, and arms

ALIGNMENT CUES & OBSTACLES
- Make sure to keep the lower body stable so that the fulcrum of the push ups emanates from the arms and shoulders, not the lower back
- Keep thinking of sitting on your heels and tucking under, using your glutes to help decompress the low back
- **Contraindications:** Some knee injuries (kneeling compresses the joint), stenosis

VARIATIONS & PEEL BACKS
- **Peel Backs:** *Thigh Stretches* on the Springboard or Cadillac. Any hip flexor stretch will help get your body ready for this exercise

IMAGINE...*you are playing peek-a-boo with the footbar.*

ELLIE SAYS...*"This is part of the Pilates X files."*

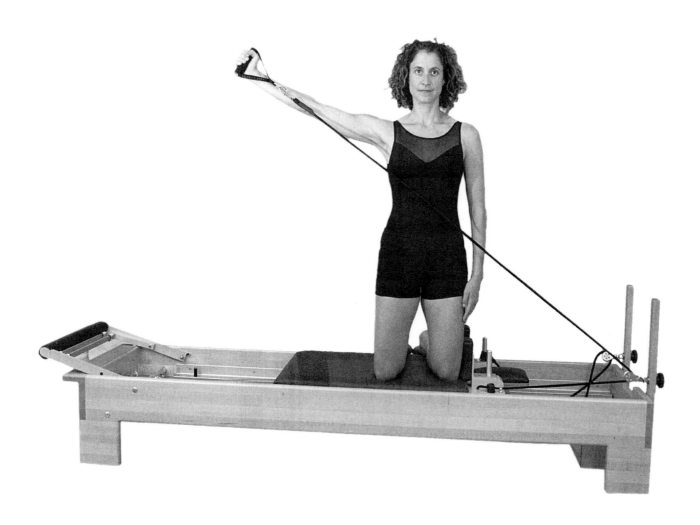

Like most Pilates exercises the Kneeling Side Arm Series is more difficult than it looks, and it is the only series that works the arms separately on the Reformer. I wasn't able to do these exercises until I got yellow springs on my Reformers because they require a huge amount of shoulder and core stability. If you're having trouble with this series you can lessen the resistance further by lengthening the straps, putting the spring bar into second gear or rising the ropes up to the top of the risers. Make sure to replace loops with handles when performing this series.

KNEELING SIDE ARM SERIES
Overhead
One Arm Rotator
Swackadee
Sidebend (Painting Under the Stairs)

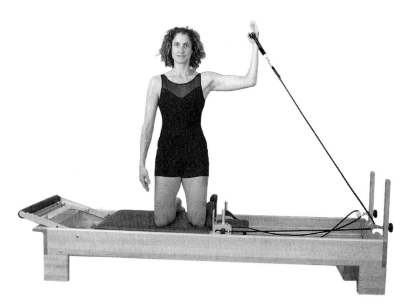

1. Starting Position—*4 to 8 repetitions*

Kneeling on carriage, facing side ways with knees directly under hips. Hand closest to risers holds handle between thumb and index finger. Arm is out to side, elbow bent to 90°, slightly in front of body, and slightly below shoulder. Palm faces toward body with fingers lengthened towards ceiling.

Inhale to prepare

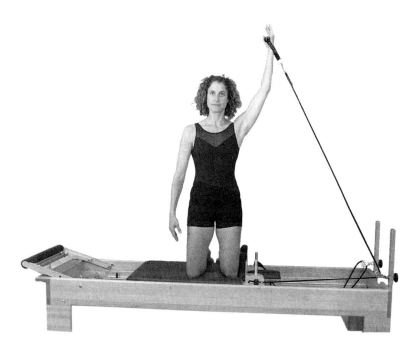

2–3. Exhale/Inhale

Exhale and you pull abdominals to spine to stabilize ribcage, engage glutes to stabilize pelvis, and raise arm straight towards ceiling, straightening elbow. Shoulder blade slides down the back as arm lifts. Inhale. Bend elbow and return to Starting Position.

MACHINE SET UP
- springs: 1 yellow, 2nd gear if necessary
- bar: N/A
- ropes: standard length or longer
- risers: down
- headrest: N/A

FUNCTIONS & TARGET MUSCLES
- Strengthens shoulder abductors
- Teaches shoulder and ribcage stability
- Works abdominals and glutes

ALIGNMENT CUES & OBSTACLES
- Raise arm from shoulder, not neck—keep scapula down as arm rises
- Do not allow body to sway, twist, or lean as carriage moves
- Keep femurs pressing forward, engaging hamstrings and glutes, and keep hips square
- Upper trap will engage as arm raises, but keep arm connected to body
- Do not lift ribs to raise arm
- Only go through ROM where scapula stay stabilized
- **Obstacles:** Tight upper traps, tight lats
- **Contraindications:** Some knee injuries (kneeling compresses the joint)

VARIATIONS & PEEL BACKS
- **Modification:** Sit in cross-legged position facing side ways if stabilizing pelvis and ribcage while kneeling is difficult or kneeling is painful
- **Modification:** If spring setting feels too challenging, lengthen rope and/or move springs into 2nd gear
- **Peel Back:** *Single Lat Pull* on Cadillac

IMAGINE...*you are the Statue of Liberty raising your torch for all to see.*

ELLIE SAYS...*"Don't lift your arm any higher than you can maintain a stable shoulder girdle. Shoulder should not rise."*

MACHINE SET UP
- springs: 1 yellow, 2nd gear if necessary
- bar: N/A
- ropes: standard length or longer
- risers: down
- headrest: N/A

FUNCTIONS & TARGET MUSCLES
- Strengthens infraspinatus, teres minor, and deltoid
- Works abdominals and glutes

ALIGNMENT CUES & OBSTACLES
- Do not open arm further to side as you straighten elbow
- Keep movements separate and precise
- Do not allow shoulder to roll in and internally rotate when returning to Starting Position
- **Contraindications:** Some knee injuries (kneeling compresses the joint)

VARIATIONS & PEEL BACKS
- **Peel Back:** *Rotator*

IMAGINE...*you are peeling your shoulder open.*

ELLIE SAYS...*"This is the best shoulder stability exercise ever...."*

1. Starting Position—*4 repetitions*
Kneeling on carriage facing side ways with knees directly under hips, next to shoulder rests. Hand closest to footbar holds handle, with elbow bent to 90° and forearm touching torso. Make a soft fist around handle with thumb on top. Fist faces the well of the Reformer (not shown).

Inhale to prepare

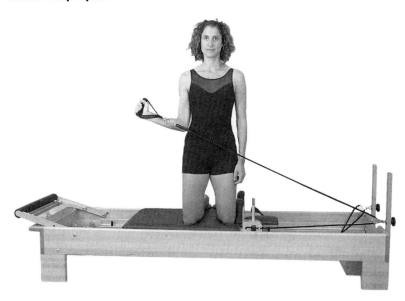

2–3. Exhale/Inhale
Exhale as you pull abdominals to spine to stabilize rib cage, engage glutes to stabilize pelvis and open forearm (externally rotate humerus) towards side to about 50–70°, keeping elbow in contact with torso. Inhale and hold.

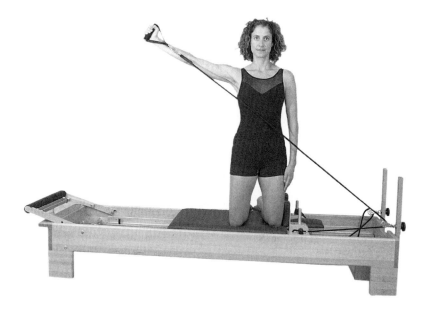

4–5. Exhale/Inhale
Exhale to pull scapula toward spine, slowly straighten elbow, punching arm to side. Inhale. Bend elbow in towards body, then internally rotate humerus to bring arm back to Starting Position.

1. Starting Position—*4 repetitions*

Kneeling on carriage facing side ways with knees directly under hips and placed next to shoulder rests. Hand closest to footbar holds handle with elbow bent and forearm resting across body, as if you're holding your stomach (not shown).

Inhale to prepare

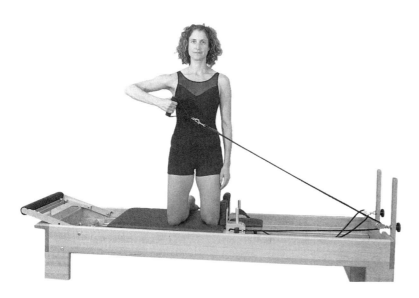

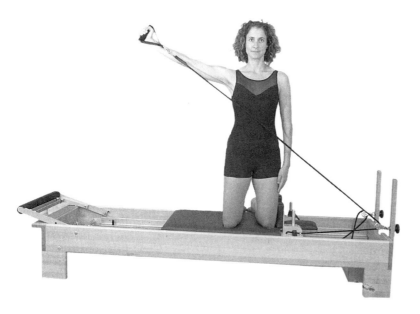

2–3. Exhale/Inhale

Pull abdominals to spine to stabilize rib cage, engage glutes to stabilize pelvis. Keeping elbow bent, pull and lift upper arm diagonally up and to the side, initiating movement from shoulder. With elbow above shoulder, keeping wrist bent, straighten elbow, making one long diagonal line. When elbow is fully extended, straighten wrist—the sword is drawn. Think: "elbow, wrist, hand." Inhale. Reverse arm motion to bring arm back to Starting Position. Bend wrist toward body, then elbow, then shoulder.

MACHINE SET UP

- springs: 1 yellow, 2nd gear if necessary
- bar: N/A
- ropes: standard length or longer
- risers: down
- headrest: N/A

FUNCTIONS & TARGET MUSCLES

- Strengthens deltoid
- Teaches shoulder stabilization with sequential movement of the arm
- Strengthens and stretches wrist

ALIGNMENT CUES & OBSTACLES

- Keep motion smooth, but make the wrist motion quick to avoid straining wrist
- "Elbow. Wrist. Hand. Hand. Wrist. Elbow." Cue it like that
- Keep femurs pressing forward, engaging hamstrings and glutes, and keep hips square
- **Contraindications:** wrist issues, Carpal Tunnel Syndrome, knee issues

VARIATIONS & PEEL BACKS

- **Peel Back:** *One Arm Rotator*

IMAGINE...*you are slowly drawing your sword out of its scabbard.*

SUSI SAYS...*"This is a great exercise for clients who play tennis and golf because it works the wrist."*

ELLIE SAYS...*"Swakadee is great exercise for stretching out the wrists after the Plank Series."*

SIDEBEND
(PAINTING UNDER THE STAIRS)

MACHINE SET UP
- springs: 1 yellow, 2nd gear if necessary
- bar: N/A
- ropes: standard length or longer
- risers: down
- headrest: N/A

FUNCTIONS & TARGET MUSCLES
- Teaches sequential movement of the arm and shoulder stabilization
- Strengthens triceps, and lats
- Stretches quadratus lumborum and obliques
- Stretches wrist

ALIGNMENT CUES & OBSTACLES
- Keep shoulders down
- Keep neck in line with curve of spine
- Humerous and shoulder don't move—think: elbow extension
- Keep hips square—squeeze glutes and push hips forward, especially the outside hip!
- **Contraindications:** unstable shoulders, sensitive knees

VARIATIONS & PEEL BACKS
- **Variation:** Start with palm facing up to work different muscles in forearm
- **Peel Backs:** *One Arm Rotator, Swakadee, Side Stretch* on Cadillac

IMAGINE...you are painting the underside of a staircase.

ELLIE SAYS...*"Make sure to keep the scapula fixed as to not over stretch your shoulder."*

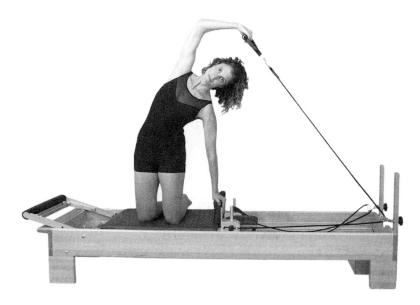

1. Starting Position—*4 repetitions*
Kneeling on carriage facing side with knees directly under hips and placed 6–10" away from shoulder rests. Bend sideways towards risers, placing one hand on the shoulder rest with fingers pointing away from body. Other hand holds handle with arm held above head and elbow bent up toward the sky. Palm is toward head.

Inhale to prepare

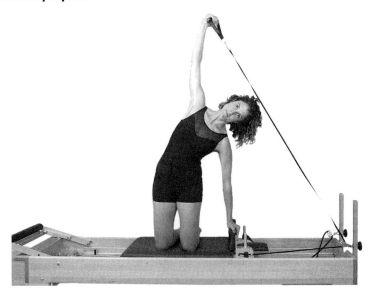

2–3. Exhale/Inhale
Maintain *Sidebend,* and keep the shoulder glued into the back as you straighten the arm overhead. Keep abdominals and glutes engaged. Inhale. Maintain *Sidebend* and reverse the motion of the arms to return to Starting Position.

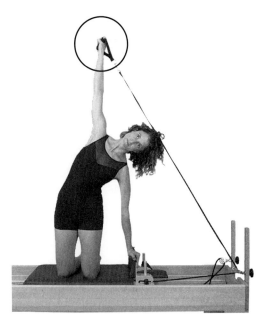

VARIATION: Painting Under the Stairs Palm Facing Up

leg series and long spine stretch

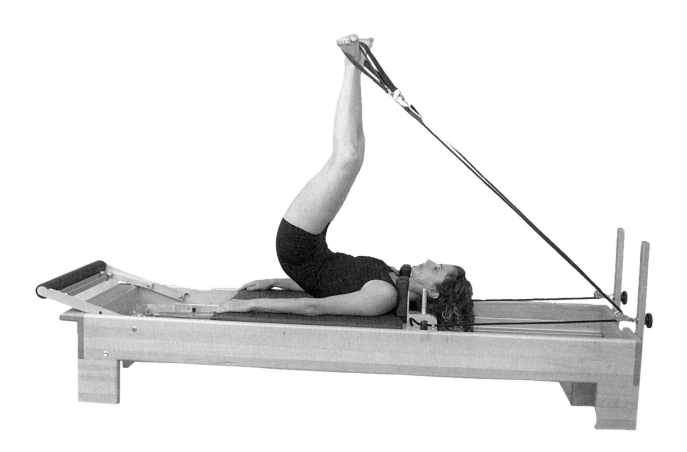

In the Leg Series, the motion of the legs challenges the stability of Neutral Pelvis/Spine while gently working the hamstrings and adductors. Work within a Range of Motion that allows for stability. As strength and stability increase, so will the Range of Motion. The parallel leg work is especially good for knee and hip rehabilitation. *Long Spine Stretch* is a loaded flexion, so be careful with any client who has disc dysfunction or osteoporosis. Don't forget to lengthen your straps before you start, and bring them back to the regular length when you're done.

LEG SERIES
Leg Pulls in Parallel
Leg Pulls in Turn Out/Turn In
Open & Close
Open & Close: Turn Out & In
Rectangles/Circles/Ovals
Hollywood Legs
Diamond Pulls
3-Way Hip Stretch

LONG SPINE
Long Spine Stretch

LEG PULLS IN PARALLEL

MACHINE SET UP

- springs: 2 red, or 1 red and 1 blue
- bar: down
- ropes: lengthened to D-ring even with shoulder rests
- risers: up or down
- headrest: up

FUNCTIONS & TARGET MUSCLES

- Teaches pelvic stability while the legs move up and down
- Strengthens hamstrings (as legs pull toward carriage), and adductors (they keep legs parallel or together when hips are in turned out position)
- Teaches disassociation of the femur from the pelvis

ALIGNMENT CUES & OBSTACLES

- Do not initiate *Leg Pulls* with back muscles—maintain Neutral Pelvis/Spine
- Keep ROM small and monitor client's Neutral Spine with a hand under the lumbar spine
- When working in parallel, keep knees bent 1–2° to avoid locking and/or hyperextending the joint
- Initiate pull from the top of the femur, not the feet—focus on medial hamstring
- For posterior pelvis: To avoid tucking pelvis, think of the pubic bone rotating down while legs return to Starting Position
- For anterior pelvis: Focus on the top of the sacrum staying connected to carriage as legs pull down—the end range of the movement is just before sacrum destabilizes
- Normal hamstring flexibility is hip flexion to 80°, so most clients will not be able to keep neutral and bring legs to 90°
- Place hand under client's lumbar spine to monitor neutral and spine extensors, and/or place hand on low abdominals to monitor client's scoop
- Keep feet relaxed—neither pointed nor flexed
- **Contraindications:** Acute phase of hamstring pull, strain, or tear

VARIATIONS & PEEL BACKS

- **Modification:** If client is small or finds maintaining neutral difficult, use 1 red & 1 blue spring (or less)
- **Modification:** To focus on pelvic stability, use thigh straps

IMAGINE... Barbie's pelvis and legs—there is no way for her pelvis to move with her legs.

ELLIE SAYS..."Parallel leg work is great for knee rehab!"

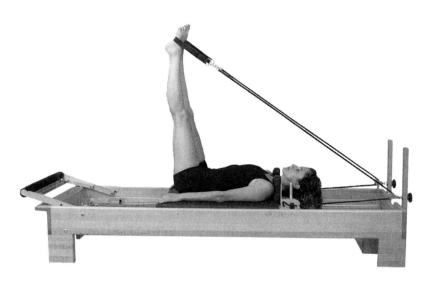

1. Starting Position—*4 to 8 reps in each position*
For Parallel: Straps around arches of feet, legs parallel with heels in line with sit bones, spine is neutral with hips in flexion. Knees are ever so softly bent. (If heels are together, knee joint cannot hyperextend).

Inhale to prepare

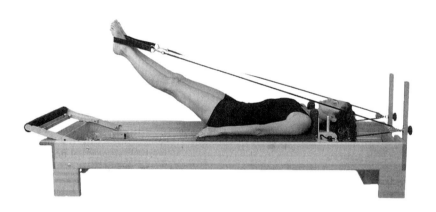

2–3. Exhale/Inhale
Engage Abdominal Scoop and pull legs down toward carriage without losing Neutral Pelvis/Spine. Focus on top of sacrum staying connected to carriage. Control back to Starting Position without tucking pelvis. Ground the coccyx into carriage.

LEG PULLS IN TURN OUT/TURN IN

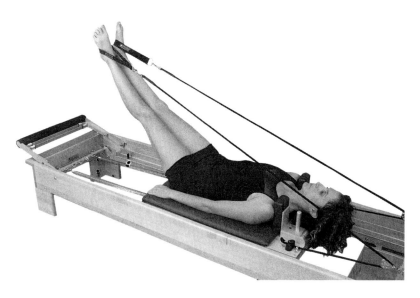

Leg Pulls in Turn Out

Leg Pulls in Turn Out
Externally rotate hips, with feet in Pilates "V"—keep heels together and knees straight. If heels are together, knee joint cannot hyperextend.

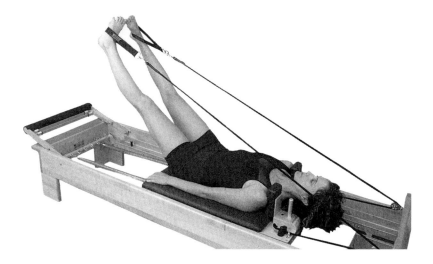

Leg Pulls in Turn In

Leg Pulls in Turn In
Start with legs in parallel, heels in line with sit bones—internally rotate femurs until toes touch (do not turn in at ankle joint).

OPEN & CLOSE

MACHINE SET UP
- springs: 2 red, or 1 red and 1 blue
- bar: down
- ropes: lengthened until D-ring is even with shoulder rests
- risers: up or down
- headrest: up

FUNCTIONS & TARGET MUSCLES
- Abdominals and deep spinal muscles stabilize pelvis and spine
- Strengthens adductors
- Teaches disassociation of the femur from the pelvis in coronal plane
- Find end ROM in the hip with a stable pelvis
- Peel back for *Leg Circles* and *Hollywood Legs*

ALIGNMENT CUES & OBSTACLES
- Keep legs at 45˚ angle through entire ROM. If legs drop and raise, the adductors aren't working against spring resistance—the carriage should move while the legs are moving
- Watch for pelvic rotation and use internal obliques to stabilize—another indicator of a rotated pelvis will be legs at different heights
- Don't tuck pelvis as legs abduct
- Tight adductors will decrease ROM in exercise, so stretch adductors before performing exercise—tight muscles are generally weak

IMAGINE..._there two large plates of glass sandwiching your feet so legs can only open and close—they can't rise._

ELLIE SAYS..._"Keep your spine and pelvis stabilized as you open your legs—this is the tricky part in this exercise."_

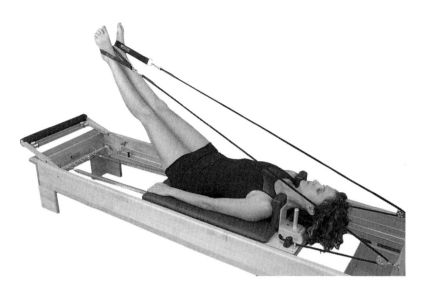

1. Starting Position—*4 to 8 repetitions*
Feet in straps with knees straight, hips in external rotation, torso stable with upper body relaxed. Hips flexed to about 45˚ without losing Neutral Pelvis/Spine.

Inhale to prepare

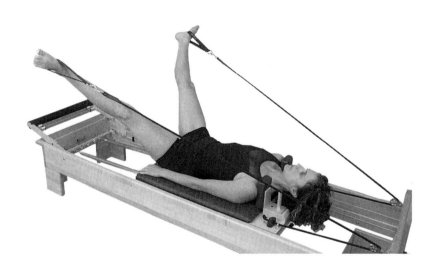

2. Exhale
Flex feet and open legs as far as possible without losing Neutral Pelvis/Spine. Carriage should move.

3. Inhale
Point feet and pull legs back to Starting Position.

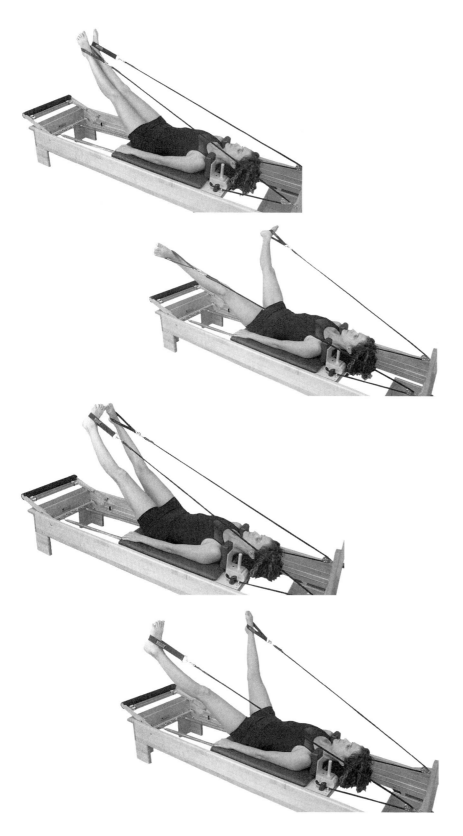

Open & Close: Turn Out & In

Open legs with hips in turn out, at end range of abduction medially rotate hip and close legs. Also do the reverse, begin with legs in medial rotation for abduction, and close legs with hip in external rotation.

Great way to lubricate the hip joints and stretch the external rotators of the hip.

Open & Close: Turn Out & In

MACHINE SET UP
- springs: 2 red, or 1 red & 1 blue
- bar: down
- ropes: lengthened until D-ring is even with shoulder rests
- risers: up or down
- headrest: up

FUNCTIONS & TARGET MUSCLES
- Strengthens hamstrings and adductors, turn out strengthens hip rotators
- Abdominals and deep spinal muscles stabilize pelvis and spine while hip moves through wide ROM
- Teaches disassociation of the femur from the pelvis as hips move in multiple planes

ALIGNMENT CUES & OBSTACLES
- ROM is greater in turn out—*Leg Circles* will be bigger than *Rectangles*
- When in parallel, focus on knees staying straight up to ceiling
- When in turn out, feel femur wrapping around to outside of legs to increase and maintain external rotation of hip. If client has unstable pelvis, keep ROM small when working in turn out
- Focus on moving from the top of the femur— closer to the body's center than the feet
- Keep movement precise and really differentiate between the right angles of the *Rectangles* and the curves of the *Circles*
- When in turn in, the ROM will be more like *Ovals* than *Circles*

VARIATIONS & PEEL BACKS
- **Peel Back:** *Leg Pulls*

IMAGINE...*your feet are the lead point of a pencil and you are drawing shapes in the air.*

ELLIE SAYS...*"No pooching when you lower or open your legs!"*

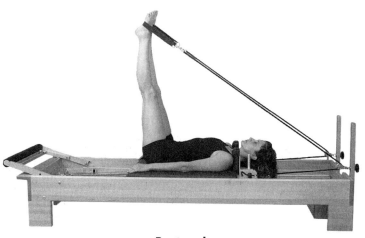

Rectangles

1. Starting Position—*4 reps in each direction*
Straps around arches of feet, legs together and parallel; spine is neutral with hips in flexion. Knees ever so softly bent.

Inhale to prepare

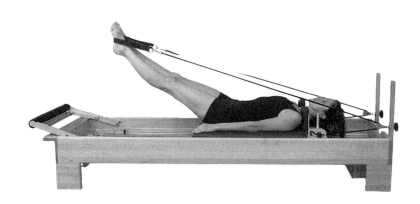

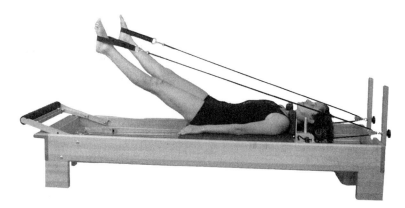

2. Exhale
Feel abdominals pull to spine keeping pelvis neutral, and pull legs down through the center and then open hip distance apart.

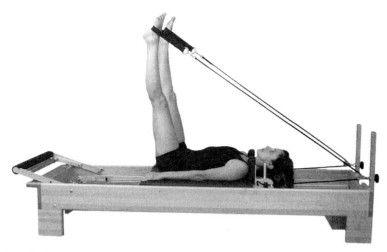

3. Inhale
Raise legs, then close them to Starting Position without losing neutral.

Repeat 4 times, then reverse directions.

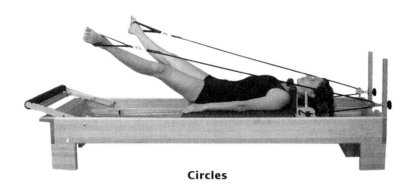

Circles

Circles
Externally rotate hip, feet in Pilates "V"—keep heels together and knees straight when moving up and down center line, inner thighs pulling together. When heels are together the knee joint cannot hyperextend.

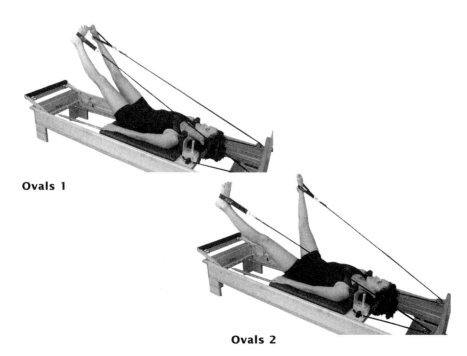

Ovals 1

Ovals
Start with legs in parallel, feet flexed, heels in line with sit bones, internally rotate femurs until toes touch (do not turn in at ankle joint).

Ovals 2

HOLLYWOOD LEGS

MACHINE SET UP
- springs: 2 red, or 1 red & 1 blue
- bar: down
- ropes: lengthened until D-ring is even with shoulder rests
- risers: up or down
- headrest: up

FUNCTIONS & TARGET MUSCLES
- Strengthens abdominals, especially the obliques, deep spinal muscles, and adductors
- Practice contralateral patterning for lower half of the body

ALIGNMENT CUES & OBSTACLES
- Always bring heels together to emphasize control and sense of center
- Keep legs moving at the same speed
- Keep ROM small to prevent straight leg from pulling pelvis into tuck position
- Keep pelvis square by using opposite internal oblique to counter the weight of straight leg pulling the pelvis away from center
- Have client put hands on pelvis (ASIS) to monitor pelvic stability
- As always, keep ROM small if client is unable to stabilize pelvis

VARIATIONS & PEEL BACKS
- **Variation:** Can perform *Hollywood Legs* as part of the Supine Series—it is more challenging to stabilize pelvis when ropes are shorter (shorter ropes with risers down intensifies the spring resistance)
- **Peel Backs:** *Frogs* and *Open & Close.* It helps to do a few *Frogs* before trying this exercise

IMAGINE...*you are performing in a Busby Berkeley movie. The camera is filming one of those great kaleidoscopic shots from above. But the camera can read the slightest instability in the pelvis. Keep your pelvis square for Busby.*

ELLIE SAYS...*"Great exercise for clients with one really weak internal oblique—they can really feel how the internal obliques work to keep pelvis from rotating."*

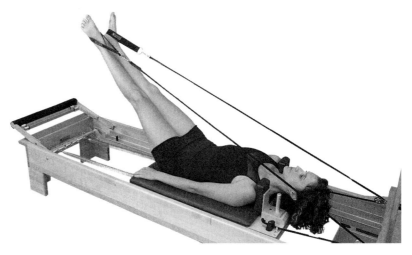

1. Starting Position—*4 to 8 repetitions (1 repetition includes both sides)*
Feet in straps with knees straight, hips in external rotation, torso stable with upper body relaxed. Hips flexed to about 45° without losing Neutral Pelvis/Spine.

Inhale to prepare

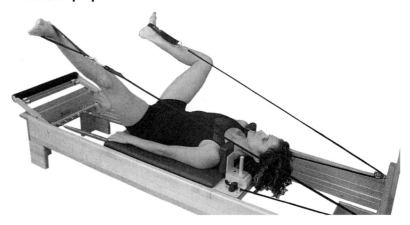

2. Exhale
Scoop abdominals to stabilize pelvis/spine and bend one leg into *Frog* position. Heel stays close to the center line of body while the other leg opens to side.

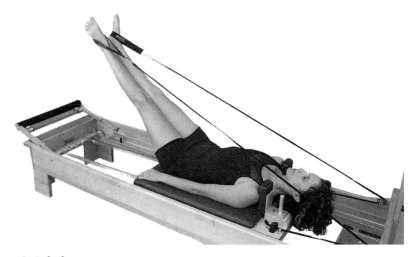

3. Inhale
Straighten leg while pulling other leg back to center with heels touching. Repeat on other side.

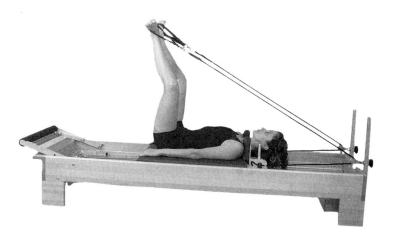

1. Starting Position—*4 to 8 repetitions*
Feet in straps with heels together, feet flexed, hips externally rotated and in flexion with knees bent open into a *Diamond* shape. Spine is neutral.

Inhale to prepare

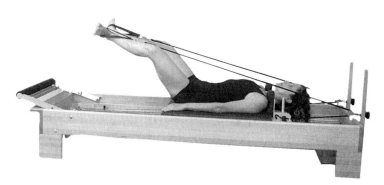

2–3. Exhale/Inhale
Exhale as you scoop abdominals and pull legs down toward carriage while keeping pelvis and spine neutral. Inhale as you control legs back to Starting Position.

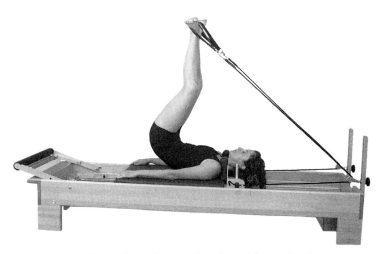

ADVANCED VARIATION: Diamond Pulls with Levitation
Put head rest down!

MACHINE SET UP
- springs: 2 red, or 1 red & 1 blue
- bar: down
- ropes: lengthened until D-ring is even with shoulder rests
- risers: up or down
- headrest: up or down

FUNCTIONS & TARGET MUSCLES
- Teaches pelvic stability while legs move up and down
- Strengthens external rotators of the hip
- Teaches disassociation of the femur from the pelvis
- The hamstring works double duty by pulling hip into extension and flexing the knee, while the biceps femoris, the lateral hamstring, works triply hard since it aids in external rotation of hip

ALIGNMENT CUES & OBSTACLES
- Leg position is halfway between *Frog* squat and straight legs
- Initiate pull from underneath the leg
- Open the knees from the back of the hip and feel the wrapping sensation around the top of the thighs
- Keep pelvis stable while initiating *Diamond Pull*—it is really easy to tuck pelvis with hips in external rotation
- Keep ROM small if client cannot maintain stability

VARIATIONS & PEEL BACKS
- **Advanced Variation:** *Diamond Pulls with Levitation:* Pull legs in *Diamond* shape down towards carriage. On an exhale engage glutes and levitate pelvis maintaining *Diamond* shape of legs. Repeat up and down motion, hinging from upper back. Caution: Make sure head rest is down when levitating!
- **Peel Backs:** *Frogs, Leg Pulls*

IMAGINE...*you're moving your legs from the panty line muscles contracting.*

ELLIE SAYS... *"This is a great exercise for creating that 'high butt' we often use as a selling point of Pilates."*

MACHINE SET UP

- springs: 2 red, or 1 red & 1 blue
- bar: down
- ropes: lengthened until D-ring is even with shoulder rests
- risers: up or down
- head rest: down

FUNCTIONS & TARGET MUSCLES

- Reinforces sequential movement of spine and concept of Levitation
- Strengthens glutes, hamstrings, and abdominals
- Stretches spinal erectors

ALIGNMENT CUES & OBSTACLES

- Do not roll up onto neck—keep weight balanced on upper back/shoulder blades
- Lengthen and stretch spine while rolling down
- Really push feet into loops on descent of pelvis
- Don't break at the hips when you roll down through the spine
- Do not tense neck or round shoulders forward while rolling up or down
- **Obstacles:** Weak glutes, tight spinal erectors, tight hamstrings
- **Contraindications:** disc dysfunction, osteoporosis, neck problems/injuries

VARIATIONS & PEEL BACKS

- **Modifications:** When rolling down through the spine, place hands on tops of thighs to maintain angle of the hip
- **Peel Backs:** *Rectangles, Levitation Vérité, Short Spine*

IMAGINE...*your spine is being pulled into, traction by an invisible force as you roll down—the force of traction is so great that your pelvis will be an inch closer to the footbar after each repetition.*

ELLIE SAYS...*"Compared to Short Spine Stretch, the Long Spine Stretch is more of an active stretch, and a more loaded stretch...careful!"*

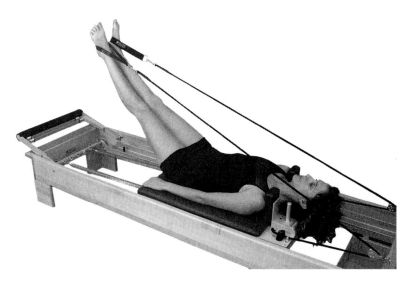

1. Starting Position—*4 repetitions (2 times each direction)*
Lying supine on carriage with feet in straps. Legs are straight and externally rotated, heels together in Pilates "V". Hips are flexed to about 45°, or to the lowest angle that Neutral Spine/Pelvis can be maintained without losing transversus engagement. The upper body is relaxed with arms resting by sides.

Inhale to prepare

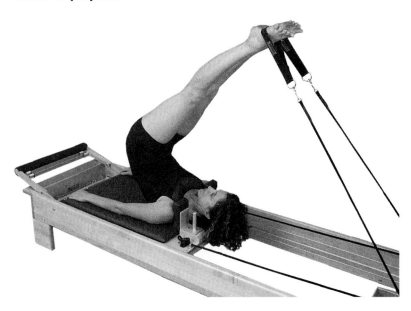

2. Exhale
Pull abdominals to spine and hinge at hips, bringing legs toward torso. When hips are flexed to 90°, engage glutes and squeeze inner thighs together to levitate pelvis into air, rolling up sequentially through spine and bringing carriage home smoothly. Weight should be balanced between scapulae, not on neck.

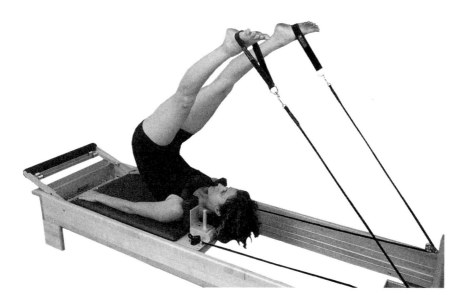

3. Inhale
Widen back and open legs to shoulder distance apart.

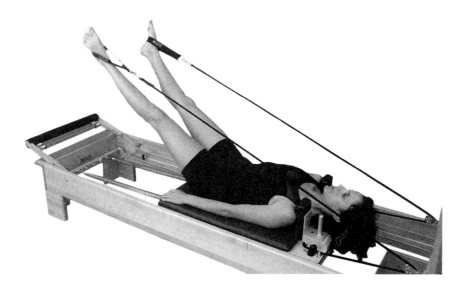

4. Exhale
Deepen abdominal engagement and articulate down, moving carriage away from home while maintaining the shape of the body—flexing only a small amount at hips to roll down sequentially through spine. Push feet into straps engaging backs of legs to facilitate hip and pelvic stability. After pelvis comes to neutral on carriage use hamstrings to pull legs down and together to Starting Position.

After 2 repetitions, reverse the positions of the legs, levitating up with legs opened to shoulder width apart, and articulating down with legs together.

BEGINNING VARIATION: Push Thighs
To take some of the load out of the back, you can press the thighs forward with your arm strength.

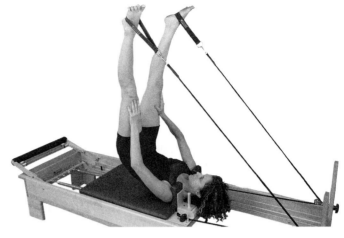

BEGINNING VARIATION: Push Thighs

ADVANCED VARIATION:
Advanced Long Spine Stretch
Stop the carriage before it hits home by levitating your hips straight up to the sky. Peel down the spine trying to maintain shape. The more you lean with your legs in front of your body, the more it becomes a control exercise and less of a stretch.

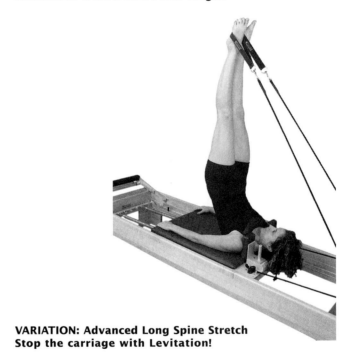

VARIATION: Advanced Long Spine Stretch
Stop the carriage with Levitation!

VARIATION: High Frog
(Advanced) From your advanced levitated position, simply bend your knees into a *Frog* squat, keeping heels together and knees as open as possible. Then, extend legs straight back up toward the sky. Repeat 5–8 times. To decrease load on spine, put hands on hips to support the weight of your body on your elbows.

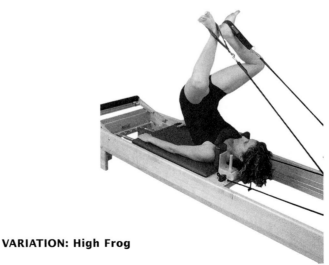

VARIATION: High Frog

1. Starting Position—*1 repetition each leg*

Lying supine on Reformer with one foot on footbar in parallel and other foot in strap with hip in as much flexion as possible while maintaining Neutral Spine/Pelvis. Both knees are straight and bottom foot is flexed.

Inhale to prepare

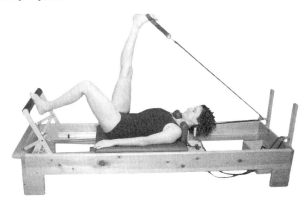

Hamstring Stretch

2. Breathing Continuously

Stay in Starting Position for 3–5 long breaths and focus on hamstrings lengthening, creating as much distance as possible between sit bones and knee. Reach through both heels to increase the stretch. To increase stretch even further, bend the standing knee while maintaining Neutral Pelvis/Spine.

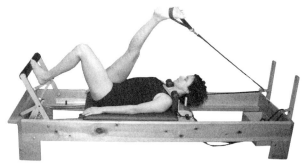

IT Band Stretch

3. Breathing Continuously

Flex foot and internally rotate the stretching leg, from the hip, then slowly cross top leg over the body as far as possible, keeping both sides of pelvis equally weighted on carriage. Keep knee straight and sickle the foot (supinate ankle) to increase stretch on lateral calf (peroneals). Hold for 3–5 long breaths.

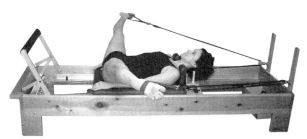

Adductor Stretch

4. Breathing Continuously

Put both feet in loops. Open legs out to side (second position in ballet), keeping both hips square. Hold stretch for 3–5 long breaths.

Switch legs and repeat Hamstring and IT Band on other side.

MACHINE SET UP

- springs: 2 red, or 1 red & 1 blue
- bar: down
- ropes: lengthened until D-ring is even with shoulder rests
- risers: up or down
- headrest: up

FUNCTIONS & TARGET MUSCLES

- Stretches hamstrings, IT Bands, and adductors

ALIGNMENT CUES & OBSTACLES

- This is similar to the *3-Way Hip Stretch* in mat work, but the strap holds the leg up so the upper body can relax
- For hamstring stretch, really focus on keeping sit bones grounded to maximize the hamstring stretch
- For IT Band stretch, focus on keeping hips square and weighting side of pelvis of stretching leg
- IT Band stretch is great for stretching the sciatic nerve

IMAGINE...*your sits bones are anchored to the mat.*

ELLIE SAYS...*"Great way to get the hips stretched."*

CONTROL FRONT

MACHINE SET UP
- springs: 1 yellow & 1 blue
- bar: high
- ropes: N/A
- risers: N/A
- headrest: N/A

FUNCTIONS & TARGET MUSCLES
- Challenges balance and coordination
- Works abdominals, glutes, calves, deltoids, lats, and pecs

ALIGNMENT CUES & OBSTACLES
- Focus on isolating the movement at shoulder or ankles
- Feel energy shooting out the top of the head—keep neck long
- Don't allow pelvis to sink—really engage the glutes and abdominals
- Keep shoulders away from ears—slide scapulae down back
- Raise leg as high as possible without hyperextending low back
- Engage adductors by squeezing inner thighs together
- **Obstacle:** Weak upper body
- **Contraindications:** Shoulder injuries, wrist issues (Carpal Tunnel, Repetitive Stress Injury)

VARIATIONS & PEEL BACKS
- **Modification:** If necessary use the "pike to *Plank*" motion to relax/stretch back in between elements
- **Peel Backs:** *Plank, Control Front* on Mat

IMAGINE...*your body is a solid Plank, and if someone were to step on your back, your body could withstand the weight.*

ELLIE SAYS...*"Everything is working here: the core, the upper body, the legs, the booty. But you still control the motion with the abdominals."*

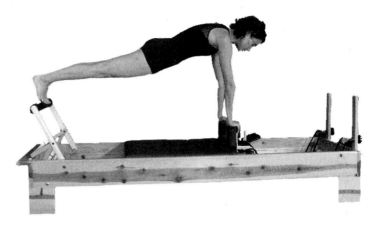

1. Starting Position—*3 with arms only, 3 with legs only, 6 full alternating sides*
Place hands on shoulder rest facing back of machine, fingers pointing towards risers. Without moving carriage, place feet on footbar. Knees will be bent at first to stay home. Feet should be in a small Pilates "V" with heels touching. Press carriage out as you come into a *Plank* position.

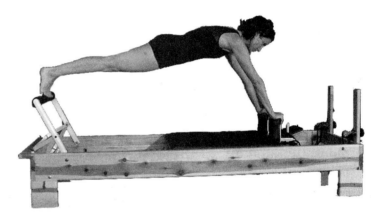

2. Breathing Continuously
Press carriage out and in from the arms maintaining *Plank* position and keeping feet still in space. The carriage moves, but the body doesn't. Come back to Starting Position each time. Repeat 3 times.

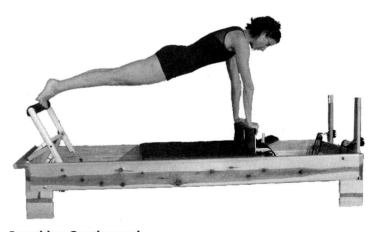

3. Breathing Continuously
Maintain *Plank* position and position of shoulders over hands while pressing carriage out and in by pointing and flexing the feet—ankles move the carriage. Keep inner thighs engaged. Repeat 3 times.

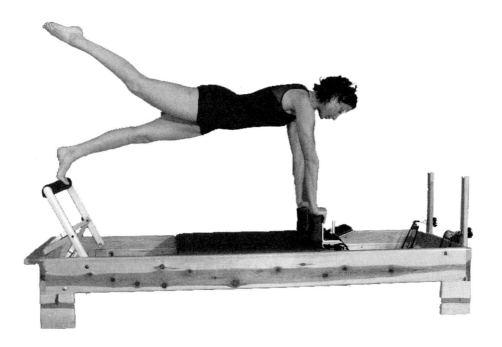

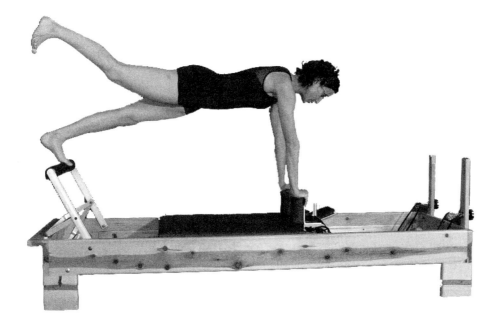

4. Breathing Continuously

Continue ankle movement as you lift right foot off bar using glute (don't hyperextend lumbar spine). Point foot as you rock forward and flex foot as you rock back (both feet point and flex simultaneously). Keep leg level as you move the carriage. Maintain alignment of shoulders over hands as carriage moves. Point/flex 3 times, then switch legs. Repeat the full exercise 3 times.

To end exercise, pike your body to bring the carriage home and step off bar onto carriage, keeping carriage still. Release hands and stretch back of body in a forward bend (bend knees if necessary). Shake head "no" and nod head "yes" to release neck.

CONTROL BACK

MACHINE SET UP
- springs: 1 yellow & 1 blue
- bar: high
- ropes: N/A
- risers: N/A
- headrest: N/A

FUNCTIONS & TARGET MUSCLES
- Strengthens triceps, lats, and hip flexors
- Works abdominals, glutes, scapula stabilizers, and adductors
- Stretches hamstrings

ALIGNMENT CUES & OBSTACLES
- Move carriage out as you lift leg—focus on inner thigh doing the lifting
- Keep shoulders down—really press heels of hand into shoulder rest and support shoulders with lats
- Maintain *Coccyx Curl* throughout exercise—super Abdominal Scoop
- Foot should be flexed at full height of leg lift to really stretch hamstring and calf
- **Contraindications:** Shoulder injuries, wrist issues (Carpal Tunnel, Repetitive Stress Injury)

VARIATIONS & PEEL BACKS
- **Variation:** Try circling leg as it comes off carriage: first out, then in
- **Peel Backs:** *Control Back & Reverse Plank* on the Mat

IMAGINE...*your leg flies up with no resistance as you send the carriage back.*

SUSI SAYS...*"It really helps your clients if you sing Control by Janet Jackson while they're performing this exercise."*

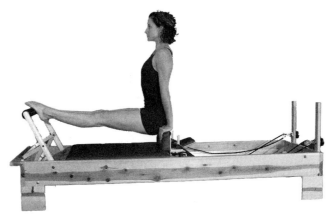

1. Starting Position—*6 times alternating sides*
Mount Reformer: hand, foot, hand, foot. Place hands on shoulder rests, fingers pointed toward pelvis, arches on footbar with feet in parallel, ankles and knees touching, and inner thighs really pull together. Round lumbar spine into *Coccyx Curl* using abdominals and engaging glutes.

Inhale to prepare

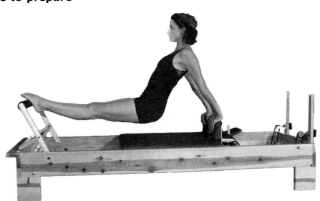

2. Exhale
Start by pressing the carriage out and in 4 times using the arms, coming back to Starting Position each time. The movement should have a smooth, rocking quality.

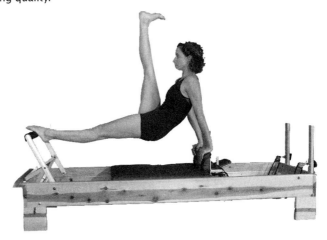

3–4. Inhale/Exhale
Inhale, maintain this rocking motion as you press carriage out, lift right foot off bar, bringing leg toward body and flexing foot. Exhale as you reach through the leg and point foot while controlling carriage back to home, and gently placing foot on bar, returning to Starting Position. Repeat 6 times, alternating sides each time.

short box series

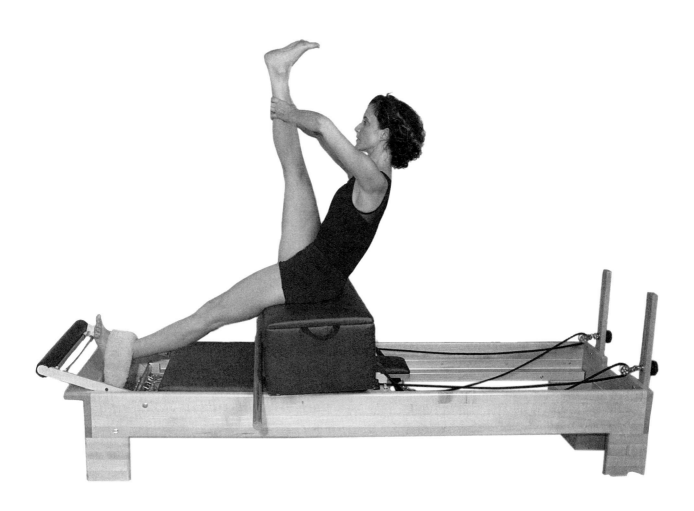

The Short Box Series is fun because you get to use the foot strap (in our studio we put a comfy fuzzy around it) that is usually tucked away and hidden under the springs. The box is placed horizontally across the carriage with the back edge flush with the shoulder rests. For clients 5'6" or taller, place the back edge of the box between the shoulder rests and pegs. (To make the box stable in this position, you may insert sticky pads under the lower edge.) Keep a pole handy in front of the box.

BEGINNING	**INTERMEDIATE**	**ADVANCED**
Round Back Roll Down	*Flat Back Hinge*	*Round Back Roll Down Variation*
Old Man at the Gym	*Twist Round Back*	*Spear a Fish/Around the World*
Twist with a Stick	*Flat Back Twist*	*Side Sit Ups/Twist & Hover*
Up & Over a Barrel	*Climb a Tree*	

ROUND BACK ROLL DOWN

MACHINE SET UP
- springs: all, in 2nd gear
- bar: down
- ropes: N/A
- risers: N/A
- headrest: N/A

FUNCTIONS & TARGET MUSCLES
- Strengthens abdominals and hip flexors
- Reinforces sequential movement of the spine
- Works hip abductors

ALIGNMENT CUES & OBSTACLES
- Keep pecs relaxed, shoulders down, and collarbones wide when rounding spine and rolling down
- Maintain leg alignment by pressing out evenly through hip, knees, and ankles
- Roll back only as far as you can control the return—don't jerk upper body to initiate roll up
- Do not jam chin into chest—Squeeze the Tangerine, don't juice it
- Feel ribs expand to sides during inhale (that's why your hands are placed there)
- **Contraindications:** disc dysfunction, osteoporosis

VARIATIONS & PEEL BACKS
- **Peel Back:** *Roll Downs*

IMAGINE...*your spine is making a capital C-Curve.*

ELLIE SAYS...*"Great for really tight clients because they finally have their hips and knees in a relaxed position."*

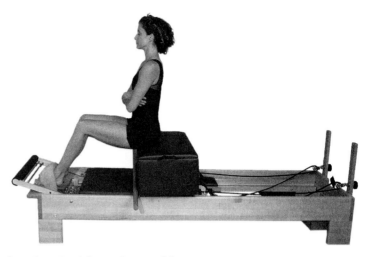

1. Starting Position—*3 repetitions*
Seated upright with sit bones placed at front edge of the box. Feet are on the wood of Reformer with parallel legs open to sides and pressing out against the foot strap. Knees are bent to 90°. Arms are criss-crossed over front of body with hands touching sides of rib cage.

Inhale to prepare

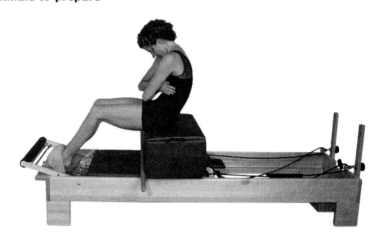

2. Exhale
Deeply contract abdominals, pulling entire spine into a full capital C-Curve.

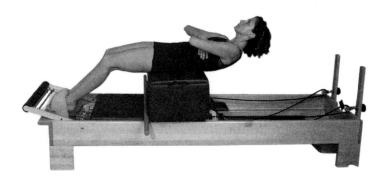

3. Inhale
Roll Down sequentially through spine, imprinting each vertebra onto the box, lengthening spine as you articulate. *Roll Down* as far as you are able to keep the transversus engaged. Keep upper back and neck in flexion.

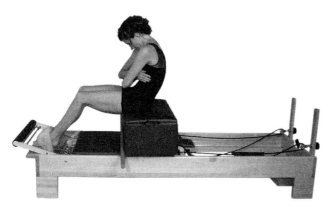

4–5. Exhale
Deepen abdominal engagement, imprinting lumbar spine onto the box, and roll up sequentially from top to bottom, ending in a full spine C-Curve.

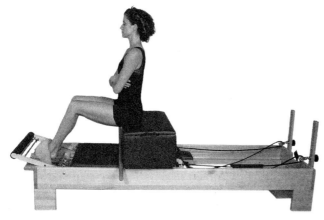

5. Inhale
Stack up from the base of the spine coming to upright posture.

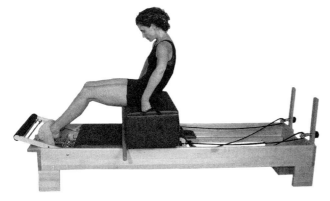

ADVANCED VARIATION: Advanced Round Back Roll Down 1

ADVANCED VARIATION:
Advanced Round Back Roll Down:
Hold on to the side handles on the box and roll all the way back into extension, allowing your head to release completely at the bottom. To return, always start by Squeezing the Tangerine, starting the ascent with the chin pulling into the chest.

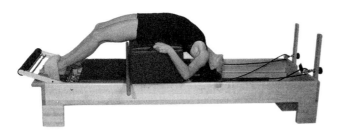

ADVANCED VARIATION: Advanced Round Back Roll Down 2

MACHINE SET UP
- springs: all, in 2nd gear
- bar: down
- ropes: N/A
- risers: N/A
- headrest: N/A

FUNCTIONS & TARGET MUSCLES
- Strengthens abdominals and hip flexors
- Works spinal erectors and scapula stabilizers
- Reinforces separation of femur from pelvis

ALIGNMENT CUES & OBSTACLES
- Keep the movement small and increase ROM as strength and body awareness increase
- Do not hyperextend lumbar spine—*Hinge* only as far as abdominals can support torso
- Keep shoulders down—remember the spine can lengthen without the shoulders rising toward the ears
- Watch for "head bobbing"—keep head stable

VARIATIONS & PEEL BACKS
- **Intermediate/Advanced Variation:** Hold a stick overhead to make the exercise more challenging

IMAGINE...*you are smelling a rose growing from your chest.*

SUSI SAYS...*"These Round and Flat Back versions of Roll Downs are wonderful abdominal exercises for clients with neck and shoulder issues because they don't need to raise their head and necks against gravity or hold onto a bar or straps."*

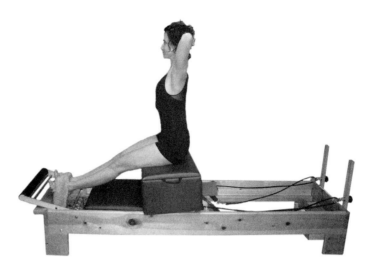

1. Starting Position—*4 repetitions*
Seated on short box with flexed feet, metatarsals hooked under foot strap. Legs are straight with hips in turn out to create a small Pilates "V" with feet. Scoot back as far as needed to feel a strong hold on the foot strap with feet. Interlace fingers behind head with elbows wide.

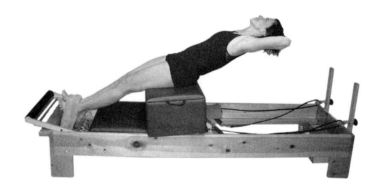

2. Inhale
Lift through spine, squeeze inner thighs together, gently engage low glutes and hinge back at hips, keeping back flat.

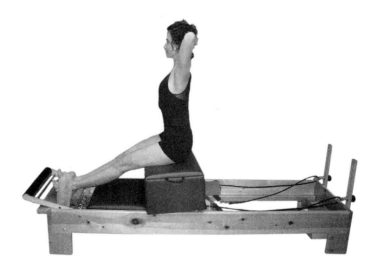

3. Exhale
Lengthen spine while hinging up to return to Starting Position, seated upright.

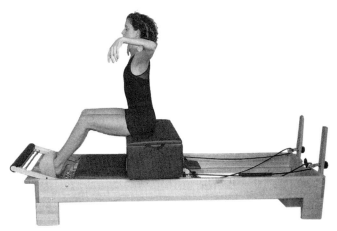

1. Starting Position—*8 sets with pulse, 8 sets without*
Seated upright with sit bones placed at front of the box. Arches are on the front edge of Reformer with parallel legs open to sides and pressing out against the foot strap. Knees are bent to 90˚. Place stick behind neck, resting on shoulders, with forearms draped over it and hands hanging in front.

Inhale to lengthen spine

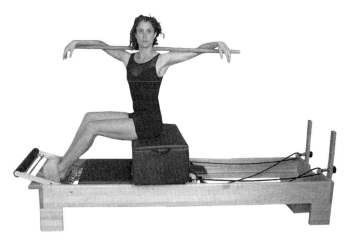

2–3. Exhale/Inhale
Exhale, keeping pelvis square, twist ribs and upper body to the right, deepen abdominal engagement and deepen twist with a small pulse. Inhale. Lengthen spine and return to center.

Repeat twisting to the left to complete the set. After 8 sets eliminate the pulse and twist smoothly alternating sides.

MACHINE SET UP
- springs: all, in 2nd gear
- bar: down
- ropes: N/A
- risers: N/A
- headrest: N/A

FUNCTIONS & TARGET MUSCLES
- Strengthens and stretches obliques and quadratus lumborum
- Teaches spinal rotation with pelvic stability
- Works abductors of hip
- *Twist with Stick* works scapula stabilizers

ALIGNMENT CUES & OBSTACLES
- Keep pelvis square and rotate the ribs
- Lengthen spine with abdominals to facilitate rotation
- Do not collapse back of neck
- Motion in the knees is symptomatic of an unstable pelvis

VARIATIONS & PEEL BACKS
- If you find yourself without a stick, perform exercise with straight arms opened out to the sides (2nd position)
- **Variation:** *Twist with Stick*: Hold the stick overhead, with arms wide facilitating scapular stabilization. Lengthen spine on inhale. Exhale and slowly rotate ribs to one side, keeping both sides long (no side bending). Keep pelvis square. Repeat 3 times alternating sides

IMAGINE...*your torso is a wet cloth and you're wringing out the excess water as you twist your waist.*

ELLIE SAYS...*"If all you got's a broom, then use a broom."*

SUSI SAYS...*"This is a great waist whittler."*

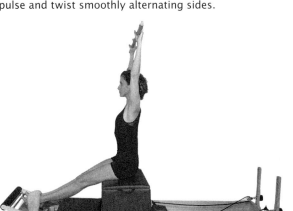

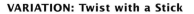

VARIATION: Twist with a Stick

MACHINE SET UP
- springs: all, in 2nd gear
- bar: down
- ropes: N/A
- risers: N/A
- headrest: N/A

FUNCTIONS & TARGET MUSCLES
- Stretches and strengthens obliques and quadratus lumborum
- Works hip abductors and scapula stabilizers
- Peel back for *Spear a Fish* and *Around the World*

ALIGNMENT CUES & OBSTACLES
- This stretch is equal parts side bending and lengthening
- Keep both sit bones in contact with box
- Keep head centered between arms—don't just move arms to side, move the spine
- Stabilize scapulae–keep shoulders away from ears

IMAGINE...*both sides of your torso are lengthening as you reach Up & Over the Barrel.*

ELLIE SAYS...*"I've got three words to say— Xena. Warrior. Princess."*

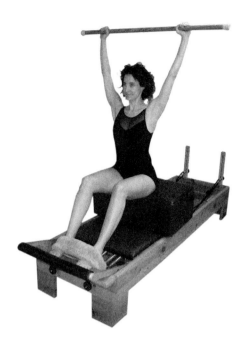

1. Starting Position—*4 repetitions each side*
Seated upright with sit bones placed at front of the box. Arches are on the front edge of Reformer with parallel legs open to sides and pressing out against the foot strap. Knees are bent to 90°. Arms hold stick overhead with hands wide to facilitate shoulder stability.

Inhale and lengthen spine

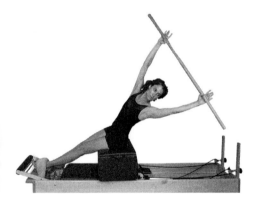

VARIATION: Flat Back Twist
(Intermediate) Here you combine three exercises: *Flat Back Hinge, Twist with Stick,* and *Up & Over a Barrel.* Start seated with stick reaching overhead (Xena Warrior Princess again), and reach stick *"Up & Over a Barrel"* and diagonally back. Keep right hip down. Continue exhaling as you rebound back to seated position, keeping scapulae sliding down the back and the shoulders away from the ears. Inhale. Lengthen spine as you come through the center and twist to the right. Repeat for 3 more sets alternating sides. Now you're ready for the challenge of *Spear a Fish.*

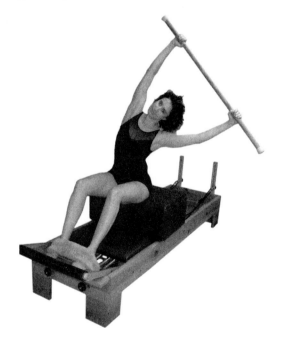

2–3. Exhale/Inhale
Exhale, as you pull abdominals to spine, lengthening spine even more, and side bend to the left without collapsing left ribs; keep left sit bones down. Inhale. Lengthen spine to return to center and prepare to side bend to the right. Repeat again only this time instead of side bending to the left, translate ribcage to the left, keeping both sides of the waist long.

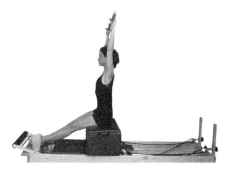

1. Starting Position—*4 repetitions each side*
Seated on short box with flexed feet hooked under foot strap. Legs are straight with hips in turn out to create a small Pilates "V" with feet. Scoot back as far as necessary, create a strong hold on the foot strap with feet. Arms are overhead, holding the stick with hands placed wide to facilitate scapular stabilization.

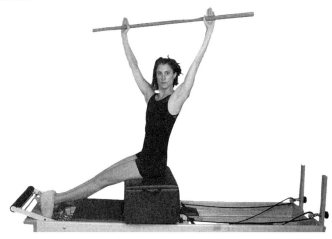

2. Inhale
Lift spine and twist spine to left, keeping pelvis square and shoulders away from ears.

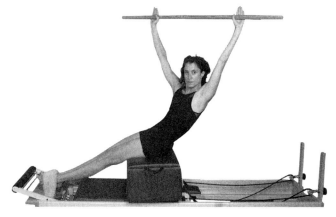

3–4. Exhale/Inhale
Exhale to pull low abdominals to spine, *Coccyx Curl* to initiate rolling down one vertebra at time, bringing left side of spine in contact with the box. Roll down only as far as the transversus remains engaged. Inhale at the bottom.

5. Exhale
Roll up sequentially, maintaining the twisted C-Curve all the way to sitting. Stack up spine from bottom to top, lengthening spine and twisting ribs to the left, keeping pelvis square.

Repeat exercise to the right, and continue alternating sides for 3 more sets.

MACHINE SET UP
- springs: all, in 2nd gear
- bar: down
- ropes: N/A
- risers: N/A
- headrest: N/A

FUNCTIONS & TARGET MUSCLES
- Strengthens abdominals, targeting the obliques
- Works adductors, quads, low glutes, and shoulder stabilizers

ALIGNMENT CUES & OBSTACLES
- If client experiences pain in low back or quadratus lumborum, have them decrease their ROM and engage transversus more
- Breaths are long and smooth to really support the movement
- Really lengthen spine to twist and curve— think: spinal stretch, not spinal compression
- Create oppositional energy in the body, up through torso and out of the feet
- **Obstacles:** Tight upper traps, weak obliques
- **Contraindications:** disc dysfunction, osteoporosis

VARIATIONS & PEEL BACKS
- If you find yourself without a stick, perform exercise with straight arms up by your ears

IMAGINE...*you are a piece of taffy being pulled in both directions.*

ELLIE SAYS...*"This is an exhilarating exercise."*

SPEAR A FISH

MACHINE SET UP
- springs: all, in 2nd gear
- bar: down
- ropes: N/A
- risers: N/A
- headrest: N/A

FUNCTIONS & TARGET MUSCLES
- Strengthens abdominals, obliques, QL, and spinal erectors
- Works adductors, quads, low glutes, hip flexors, and shoulder stabilizers

ALIGNMENT CUES & OBSTACLES
- Keep both sides long—do not collapse rib cage
- "Lift. Twist. Spear."
- Every inhale is an opportunity to lengthen the spine, and every exhale to deepen Abdominal Scoop
- Head stays centered between arms—don't just move arms to the floor, hinge at hips, bringing torso toward floor
- **Contraindications:** disc dysfunction, osteoporosis

VARIATIONS & PEEL BACKS
- Start by teaching with airplane arms first and assist client by holding their hand to help lift up body to side position—progress to *Spear a Fish*
- **Peel Back:** *Flat Back Twist*

IMAGINE...*you are diving into water to spear a fish but your legs anchor you in the boat, your toes tucked under the bench in front of you.*

ELLIE SAYS...*"Keep your spine in slight flexion...we want to work the obliques not the QL's. If that's too jargon-y, I'm talkin' about y'alls backs."*

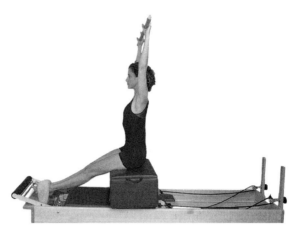

1. Starting Position—*4 repetitions each side*
Seated on short box with flexed feet hooked under foot strap. Legs are straight with hips in turn out to create a small Pilates "V" with feet. Scoot pelvis back as far as necessary to feel a strong hold on the foot strap with feet. Arms are overhead holding the stick with hands placed wide to facilitate scapular stabilization.

Inhale and lift spine and twist rib cage to left, keeping pelvis square and shoulders away from ears

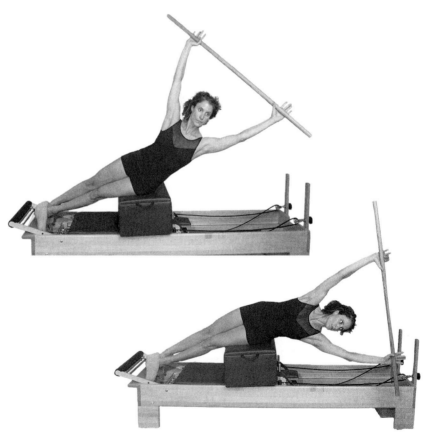

2. Inhale
Lengthen spine and fire the right glute to lift right hip and twist rib cage to left, rolling to left hip, keeping spine long and shoulders away from ears. Allow right foot to stack on top of left foot. *Spear a Fish* to the left side, by side bending from torso. Keep stick in frame around head.

3. Exhale
Lift entire upper body to pull "spear" out of the water, ending seated upright in Starting Position. Repeat starting to the right.

Continue after Steps 1 and 2 of Spear a Fish.

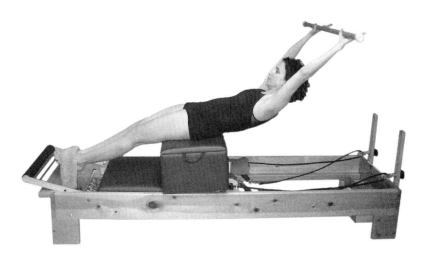

3. Exhale
From *Spear A Fish* movement, pull abdominals deeply to spine, untwist body until centered on the box with sacrum deeply imprinted and lumbar spine flexed. Arms remain overhead.

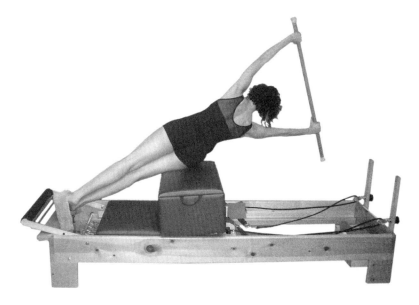

4. Inhale
Roll onto right hip, allowing feet to move in the footbar to the right. *Spear a Fish* to the right. Pausing in this position for a moment—feel the length in the spine with torso suspended over the Reformer.

5. Exhale
Lift entire upper body to pull "spear" out of the water, ending seated upright in Starting Position. Repeat starting to the right.

MACHINE SET UP
- springs: all, in 2nd gear
- bar: down
- ropes: N/A
- risers: N/A
- headrest: N/A

FUNCTIONS & TARGET MUSCLES
- Strengthens the abdominals, especially obliques and QL
- Challenges control
- Works quads, adductors, dorsiflexors, and scapula stabilizers

ALIGNMENT CUES & OBSTACLES
- Allow feet to move from side to side in the foot strap as torso moves
- Find a balance between using momentum and controlling it
- Keep lumbar spine in small amount of flexion when rolling through center (and really initiate the rolling with the abdominals, coordinating with the exhalation)
- Think of the body as one unit while rolling—legs, pelvis, ribcage, shoulders, and head all roll and twist as one
- Keep head slightly forward as you roll through center to avoid overloading the low back
- Keep stick "framing" the head—don't move from arms
- **Contraindications:** disc dysfunction, osteoporosis

VARIATIONS & PEEL BACKS
- **Modification:** To reduce challenge to shoulder stabilizers and abdominals, use airplane arms if necessary
- **Peel Back:** *Spear a Fish* should be learned first before attempting *Around the World*

IMAGINE...*your body is a hurricane with your feet as the eye of the storm.*

ELLIE SAYS...*"This is one of the rare Pilates exercises which allows the use of momentum. Have fun, but don't forget to remain in control of the motion."*

CLIMB A TREE

MACHINE SET UP
- springs: all, in 2nd gear
- bar: down
- ropes: N/A
- risers: N/A
- headrest: N/A

FUNCTIONS & TARGET MUSCLES
- Stretches hamstrings
- *Roll Down* stretches hip flexors and works abdominals
- Strengthens spinal erectors

ALIGNMENT CUES & OBSTACLES
- Straightening the leg, use biceps to pull femur into body, increasing hamstring stretch
- Keep pelvis as square as possible while stretching and rolling down
- Don't lean back to initiate *Roll Down*, use abdominals to round lumbar spine
- Roll back only go as far as you can control the roll up—increase ROM as strength increases
- Protect lumbar spine—REALLY keep transversus engaged
- Keep lumbar spine straight while stretching leg—lean torso back if necessary to avoid lumbar flexion (which really loads the spine)
- Spot client during the *Roll Down* in case extra support is required
- Keep shoulders "ka-chunked" down the back—don't let them roll forward as you hold leg
- **Obstacles:** Tight hamstrings, weak abdominals
- **Contraindication:** Disc dysfunction, osteoporosis

VARIATIONS & PEEL BACKS
- **Modification:** If tight hamstring inhibits rolling down, allow knee of top leg to soften a bit
- **Peel Back:** *Round Back Roll Downs*

IMAGINE...*your thigh is the trunk of the tree and your toes are the high branches.*

ELLIE SAYS...*"This may be the single best exercise to change the length of the hamstrings while strengthening the low back and psoas—great for tuckers!"*

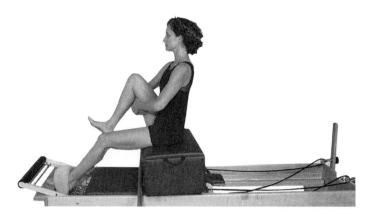

1. Starting Position—*3 stretches & 1 Roll Down*
Seated on box with one leg straight and flexed foot hooked under foot strap. The other leg is bent over forearm with hand in a fist. Opposite hand holds wrist. Spine is straight and neutral. Shoulders are open and scapulae pulled down the back.

Inhale to prepare

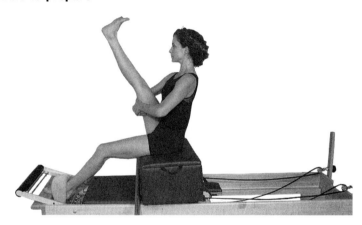

2–3. Exhale/Inhale
Exhale as you pull abdominals to spine, flex foot while straightening knee to lengthen hamstring, engage quadriceps to straighten leg, keeping pelvis square and spine straight. Do not round lumbar spine. If necessary, lean back a bit to maintain Neutral Spine. Inhale to bend knee back to Starting Position. Repeat steps 2 & 3 twice.

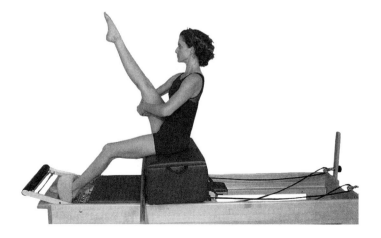

4. Breathing Continuously
On third repetition, with knee straightened, point and flex the ankle 3 times. Then circle ankle 3 times each direction. Bend knee back to Starting Position.

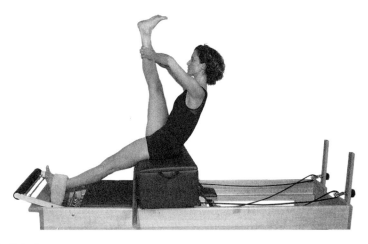

5. Exhale
Straighten leg one more time. Walk the hands up the leg as if you were climbing a tree. Holding calf, pull femur into torso to increase hamstring stretch, using biceps and bending elbows to the sides.

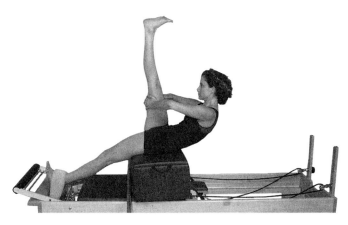

6–7. Inhale/Exhale
Inhale to lengthen spine and maintain stretch. Exhale as you pull low abdominals to spine and walk hands back down the "tree" leg as you *Roll Down* sequentially through the spine. Hands hold upper thigh with fingers interlaced; roll only as far as transversus remains engaged. Keep sacrum in contact with box as you unfurl, with heel of flexed foot reaching up.

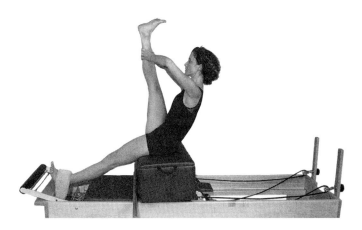

8–9. Inhale/Exhale
Inhale to prepare to roll up. Exhale, round head and neck forward and begin to roll up sequentially from top of spine to sacrum—press thigh away to assist roll up. Stack the spine as you walk hands back up the "tree" and pull leg toward your torso for one last hamstring stretch.

SUPER ADVANCED VARIATION:
Back Bend
After rolling down, release leg and reach both arms back to hold tracks of Reformer. This deepens the hip flexor stretch and increases work for the abdominals both in stabilizing the stretch and initiating the roll up. Don't allow leg to lower when reaching back

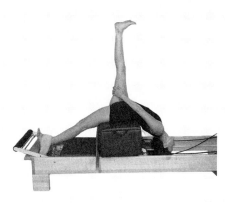

Back Bend 1

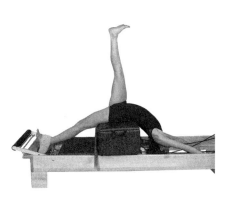

Back Bend 2

MACHINE SET UP

- springs: all, in 2nd gear
- bar: down
- ropes: N/A
- risers: N/A
- headrest: N/A

FUNCTIONS & TARGET MUSCLES

- Strengthens obliques and QL

ALIGNMENT CUES & OBSTACLES

- Keep leg as externally rotated as possible to avoid overworking TFL
- Allow head and neck to follow line of spine
- As always, keep shoulders away from ears

VARIATIONS & PEEL BACKS

- **Modification:** Arms in airplane position
- **Variation:** *Twist & Hover.* Inhale and side bend toward the well. Exhale, pull abdominals up to spine, twisting upper body toward floor. Inhale, lower torso to floor while maintaining and possibly even deepening the twist. Exhale and pull abdominals into spine to hover and raise torso. Inhale and untwist torso, ending in deep side bend. Exhale, use obliques and QL to bring torso up, returning to Starting Position
- **Peel Back:** *Up & Over a Barrel*

IMAGINE...*you are trying to pick up a cashmere scarf you dropped into the well of the Reformer. If you just lengthen the spine a little bit more you'll be able to grab it.*

ELLIE SAYS...*"The Twist & Hover variation is really fun and feels like an early modern dance exercise. Really focus on the abdominals initiating the movement. It's a channel Martha Graham moment."*

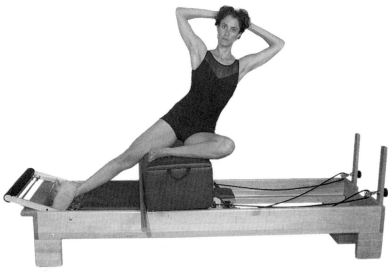

1. Starting Position—*3 to 5 repetitions*
Seated on box facing side with one leg under foot strap, foot flexed and hip externally rotated with knee toward the ceiling. The outside of the other leg rests on the box with knee bent and hip opened to the side. Spine is straight and hands are behind head with elbows wide.

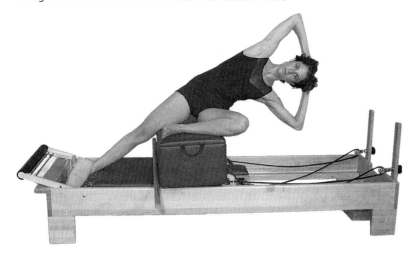

2. Inhale
Bend sideways toward well of Reformer (think: *Up & Over a Barrel*).

3. Exhale
Pulling abdominals deeply to spine, reach rib cage to pelvis to return to Starting Position.

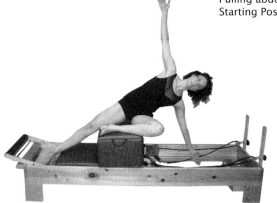

VARIATION: Twist & Hover 1

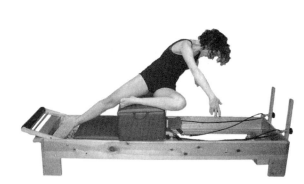

VARIATION: Twist & Hover 2

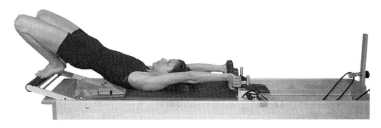

1. Starting Position—*3 repetitions in each direction*
Lying supine on carriage with feet in Pilates "V" on footbar (use a sticky pad) with hands on the shoulder rests with fingers facing out. Lift torso slightly off carriage and push carriage away until elbows are straight. Carriage will move away from home. Use abdominals and glutes to *Bridge* up sequentially, starting with tailbone until weight is balanced between scapulae—not on neck.

Inhale to prepare

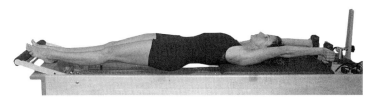

2. Exhale
Keeping pelvis high, push carriage out until knees are straight (or almost straight).

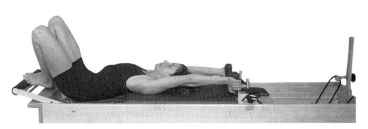

3. Inhale
Peel spine down sequentially from top to bottom, allowing pelvis to come below carriage; bend knees and move carriage toward home.

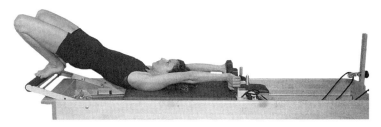

4. Exhale
As you approach home, begin to *Coccyx Curl* and continue lifting pelvis up, returning to Starting Position.

Repeat twice more, then reverse the motion—pushing carriage out with pelvis low, bridging up with straight legs, coming home with pelvis high, lowering pelvis into springs to repeat.

MACHINE SET UP
- springs: 2 red (the outer springs)
- bar: down or low with sticky pad
- ropes: N/A
- risers: N/A
- headrest: N/A

FUNCTIONS & TARGET MUSCLES
- Articulates spine and releases lumbar spine
- Works glutes, hamstrings, and deltoids
- Stretches quads

ALIGNMENT CUES & OBSTACLES
- Maintain leg alignment with knees aimed over second toes
- Lower pelvis fully into springs when rolling down—that's why you're using the outside springs
- Do not lock elbows or hunch shoulders up by ears
- Use just a little turn out at the hips—don't wrench hips open or splay the knees
- Really engage the abdominals to support spine and engage glutes to support the pelvis throughout exercise
- Feel free to keep slight amount of flexion in knees when pelvis is off carriage to decrease lumbar compression
- Really lead with the tailbone to start *Bridge,* working lumbar spine through full ROM extension to flexion
- **Contraindications:** Knee injuries, disc dysfunction, lumbar arthritis, osteoporosis, wrist or shoulder injuries

VARIATIONS & PEEL BACKS
- **Modification:** If 1st position compresses knee joints, place arches at edges of footbar (2nd position) or decrease ROM only bending knees slightly
- **Modification:** If client has tight shoulders, place hands high on hold shoulder rests
- **Modification:** To challenge ROM of entire exercise, or if client is under 5'2", use low bar setting
- **Variation:** Try rolling up with spinal flexion and lower pelvis in neutral, separating femurs from pelvis
- **Variation:** *Quad Stretch*: with pelvis high at end of exercise, place hands above client's knees and gently pull legs out toward you to stretch quads
- **Peel Backs:** *Bottom Lift, Snake & Reverse*

IMAGINE...*you are drawing a circle with your pelvis in space.*

ELLIE SAYS...*"We think Mr. Pilates tossed back a few before he came up with this one."*

TENDON STRETCH

MACHINE SET UP
- springs: 2 red or 1 red & 1 blue or yellow, (the heavier the easier to return)
- bar: high
- ropes: N/A
- risers: N/A
- headrest: N/A

FUNCTIONS & TARGET MUSCLES
- Strengthens abdominals
- Stretches spinal extensors, hamstrings and calves
- Works lats, pecs, triceps, and hip flexors

ALIGNMENT CUES & OBSTACLES
- Spot clients by holding their hips, helping them feel the "up" motion of the pelvis
- Think: head to knees to come up—keep back of neck long and jaw relaxed
- Stay as tight as possible in the pike position— if you don't your booty will hit the foot bar (ouch!)
- Fold the body in half and focus on abdominals creating the crease
- Do not hyperextend the elbows
- Stretch wrists gently into flexion before and after performing this exercise
- **Obstacles:** Tight hamstrings and/or back extensors, weak lats, weak abdominals
- **Contraindications:** Wrist and/or shoulder issues, disc dysfunction, osteoporosis

VARIATIONS & PEEL BACKS
- **Modification:** If you're experiencing difficulty bringing carriage back home, add springs
- **Modification:** Decrease spring resistance for smaller clients or to increase abdominal challenge

IMAGINE...*you're a gymnast showing off your fancy pike moves and strong arms.*

ELLIE SAYS...*"Fold in half like a hairpin."*

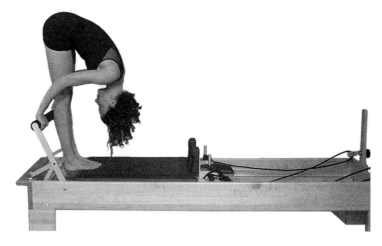

1. Starting Position—4 repetitions
Sit on footbar with hands on either side of pelvis. Place feet together in the center of the carriage with heels hanging off edge (put a sticky pad on carriage). Press heels of hands into footbar, straighten knees and bend in half at the waist into a deep pike position.

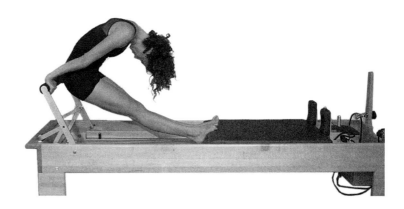

2. Inhale
Maintain pike position as much as possible, push carriage away from home by dropping down through heels (there's your *Tendon Stretch)* and bring pelvis down through arms—elbows remain straight.

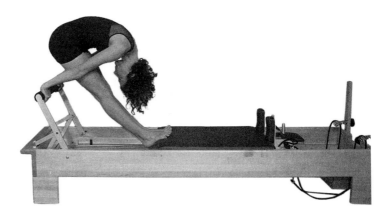

3. Exhale
Pull your abdominals to the sky, push heels of hands into footbar and return to Starting Position.

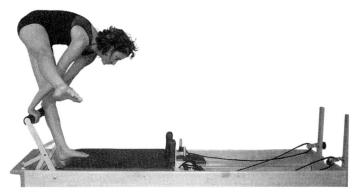

1. Starting Position—*3 repetitions each side, each position*
Sit on footbar and place left hand outside of pelvis and right hand between legs. Place left arch on the carriage with heel hanging off edge (put a sticky pad on carriage) and right leg lifted to the side in parallel. Straighten left knee and fold body in half.

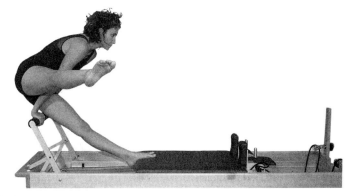

2. Inhale
Keeping elbows straight, push carriage away from home by dropping heel downward, maintaining body position.

3. Exhale
Pull abdominals to sky, push heels of hands into footbar and bring carriage home maintaining body position.

Continue with leg to the side for 3 repetitions, then circle leg around to the back for *Arabesque* version, without lowering pelvis to footbar (that's what Pilates called *Around the World*).

MACHINE SET UP
- springs: 1 red & 1 yellow, blue or red (the heavier the easier to return)
- bar: high
- ropes: N/A
- risers: N/A
- headrest: N/A

FUNCTIONS & TARGET MUSCLES
- Leg to side: strengthens TFL, glutes medius and minimus
- Leg to back: strengthens glutes of back leg and stretches hamstring of front leg
- Works abdominals, hip flexors, lats, pecs, and triceps

ALIGNMENT CUES & OBSTACLES
- Leg to back: Use glute max to maintain level of back leg, trying to create the splits as carriage moves away from home—keep back leg as high as possible
- Single leg variations are not as extreme in ROM as double leg—the motion is not about folding in half
- With leg to the side the motion has a seesaw quality
- Keep knees straight but not locked
- Keep shoulders away from ears and scapulae stabilized
- Keep neck long—do not crunch back of neck, think that the head is part of the spine
- To spot leg to back: hold onto client's leg and help them keep the leg lifted as they descend and rise—like you're pumping an oil well...

VARIATIONS & PEEL BACKS
- **Peel Backs:** *Tendon Stretch, Plank Arabesque*

IMAGINE...*your free leg uses the momentum of the upswing to transition from side to front and visa versa.*

ELLIE SAYS...*"This exercise reminds me of a man's gymnastic routine on the horse."*

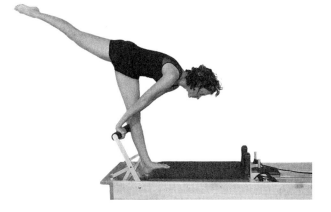

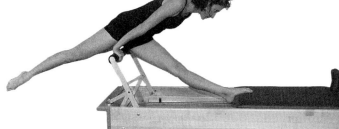

4. Breathing Continuously
Keeping your back leg really reaching up to the sky, push the carriage out, then control carriage back to home.

PRANCING

MACHINE SET UP
- springs: 2 red & 1 blue
- bar: low or high
- ropes: N/A
- risers: N/A
- headrest: up

FUNCTIONS & TARGET MUSCLES
- Strengthens and stretches plantar flexors and dorsiflexors
- Works abdominals and multifidi
- Teaches ankle alignment through entire ROM of joint

ALIGNMENT CUES & OBSTACLES
- Do not pop knees to straight—be gentle with ankle and knee joints
- Do not allow femur to internally rotate when lowering heel—work low glutes
- Keep weight evenly distributed between big and little toes—do not allow ankles to roll in or out
- Do not hyperextend the knee while straightening leg
- Keep pelvis stable—no tucking, no rocking from side to side
- Remember, only one knee bends at a time
- Always accent the "up" motion

VARIATIONS & PEEL BACKS
- Once the alternating pattern has been mastered, speed up the motion and continue breathing circularly, using every exhale to deepen abdominal engagement

IMAGINE...*your legs are made out of taffy–very stretchy–lengthening and contracting with no hard edges.*

ELLIE SAYS...*"Keep those hips stable. No samba dancing!"*

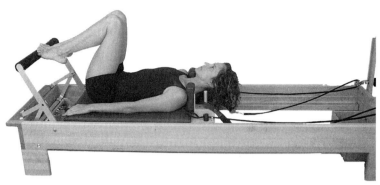

1. Starting Position—*30 prances alternating*
Lying supine on carriage with shoulders against shoulder rests, feet are parallel with the metatarsals on the footbar and heels high (relevé). Arms are resting by sides. Pelvis and spine are neutral.

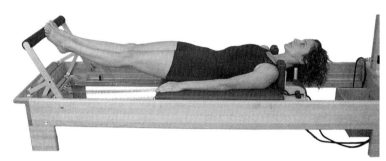

2. Inhale
Keeping heels high, press carriage away from home until legs are straight.

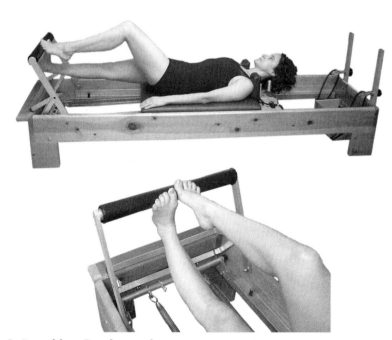

3. Breathing Continuously
Stabilize pelvis with abdominals; lower one heel under the bar while bending the other knee straight up to the ceiling, pressing the ball of the foot into the bar to make a "forced arch" (lift the heel).

4. Breathing Continuously
Smoothly return both feet to relevé position, straightening both knees.

Alternate sides.

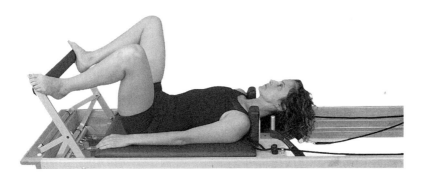

1. Starting Position—*8 to 10 repetitions*
Lying on back with arches placed at the corners of the footbar. Arms are relaxed and resting by sides.

Inhale wide through ribs to prepare

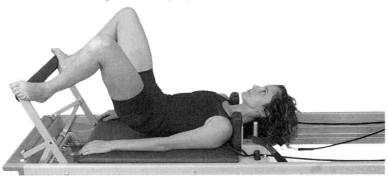

2. Exhale
Coccyx Curl and raise pelvis just off the carriage, flexing lumbar spine using abdominals and squeezing glutes.

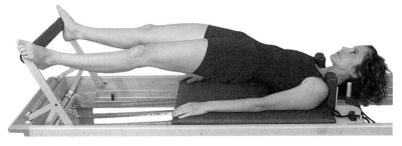

3. Inhale
Feel abdominals pull toward spine and push carriage out until knees are almost straight.

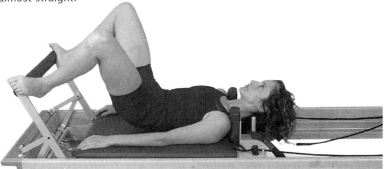

4. Exhale
Squeeze glutes and control carriage back home keeping pelvis stable and level in space.

Repeat 10 times then return home and *Coccyx Curl* down without moving the carriage.

MACHINE SET UP
- springs: 2 reds & 1 blue
- bar: low or high
- ropes: N/A
- risers: N/A
- headrest: up or down

FUNCTIONS & TARGET MUSCLES
- Strengthens hamstrings and glutes
- Works abdominals and, in turn out positions, the external rotators of the hips
- With pelvis high, works dorsiflexors and spinal erectors

ALIGNMENT CUES & OBSTACLES
- Reach knees towards feet to make space for the pelvis to rise
- Focus on abdominals when pushing carriage out on exhale, and focus on the glutes squeezing and controlling carriage home on inhale
- Do not push out all the way to straight legs if doing so jams the low back and knees
- Do not pop your ribs to the ceiling—engage upper abdominals to avoid hyperextending the spine
- Keep the inner thighs working so knees don't splay open in turn out positions
- Remember to use accordion breathing on inhale—ribs move wide, not up (which overextends thoracic spine)

VARIATIONS & PEEL BACKS
- **Modification:** Lighter spring resistance increases hamstring work
- **Peel Backs:** *Second Position Footwork, Coccyx Curls, Bridges*

IMAGINE...your abdominals are pulling the pelvis off the carriage.*

ELLIE SAYS...*"This exercises comes in handy in the sack."*

BOTTOM LIFT VARIATIONS

VARIATIONS

On Heels in 2nd Position: (Beginning)
Place heels of flexed feet on corners of footbar, raise the pelvis into a full *Bridge* (either sequentially through spine or press pelvis up maintaining neutral) and maintain height of pelvis while pushing carriage out, almost straightening legs, and controlling carriage to home. Keep pelvis stable and level in space.

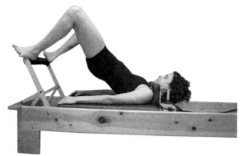

On Heels in 2nd Position

Arches in Parallel: (Beginning)
Place arches on bar with feet in parallel, ankles and knees touching (feel adductors working). Lift pelvis just barely off mat, then push carriage 3–5" from home and pulse carriage toward home in a 1–2" range, with accent on "in."

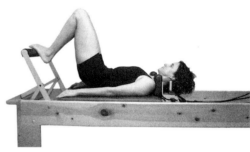

Arches in Parallel—Pulse Carriage with Accent on "In"

Single Leg on Arches: (Intermediate)
Place both heels on bar, *Bridge* three quarters of the way up and then lift one leg, bringing heel to ceiling. Press out halfway, then bring carriage home, lowering leg to level of opposite thigh. Maintain level pelvis and proper alignment throughout exercise. This exercise can also be done on heels to increase glutes and decrease hamstring work.

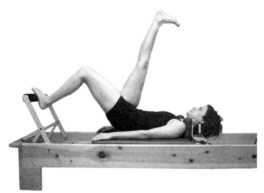

Single Leg on Arches 1

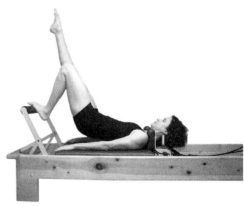

Single Leg on Arches 2

Snake and Reverse: (Beginning)
Place heels on bar in Pilates First Position, *Bridge* up without moving carriage and push carriage from home until knees are almost straight. Keeping carriage still, flex at hips to lower pelvis down to carriage to neutral position. Repeat 4 times, then reverse directions: push out—*Bridge* up sequentially, keeping pelvis high bring carriage home—crease at hips, lowering pelvis to neutral.

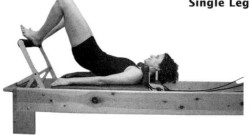

Snake and Reverse

split series

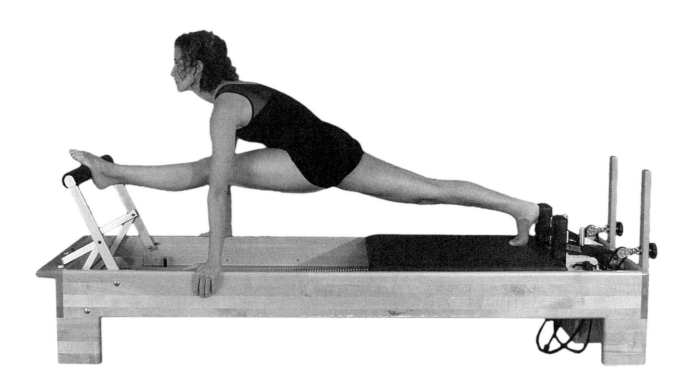

The Split Series is a great way to integrate concepts learned and perfected while lying on your back—but into standing movements. Remember, Joe Pilates was a gymnast, and splits are essential to gymnastics. These exercises focus on stretching the hips while controlling the movement of the carriage with the same muscles—creating active stretching, which stays with you.

FRONT SPLITS	**SIDE SPLITS**	**BACK SPLITS**
4-Part Stretch	*Side Splits*	*Back Splits*
Front Splits	*Bonnie Blair*	
	Speed Skating	

MACHINE SET UP

- springs: 1 blue or 1 red; less weight works adductors, more weight works abductors
- bar: down with footplate installed
- headrest: N/A

FUNCTIONS & TARGET MUSCLES

- Strengthens hip abductors and adductors
- Works abdominals and in turn out the external rotators of the hip
- Teaches/reinforces standing posture

ALIGNMENT CUES & OBSTACLES

- Perform the first 2 to 3 repetitions with hands on hips to feel alignment
- Do not allow ankles to roll in—keep arches up and lifted
- Watch rib alignment when raising arms to sides—do not allow ribs to fall behind plumb line
- Engage pelvic floor when closing the legs— think of zipping up the middle
- Keep weight evenly distributed between both feet with pelvis level and centered
- Keep weight slightly forward—don't lean back
- To increase difficulty, widen stance, placing foot on carriage closer to head rest
- Don't do this exercise if you have an unstable SI joint
- Careful if you're pregnant! Keep ROM small
- **Contraindications:** SI joint instability

VARIATIONS & PEEL BACKS

- **Variation:** Perform *Side Splits* in turn out
- **Variation:** *Pick a Flower.* With carriage as far from home as you can maintain Neutral Spine/Pelvis, bend at hips with a flat back (no flexion of spine) and reach one arm forward as if you were *Picking a Flower*—the carriage should not move while bending, "picking," or returning to standing. Repeat the action and *Pick a Flower* with the other hand. (Note to modern dancers: It should feel like a Cunningham or Horton exercise)
- **Advanced Variation:** If you have the flexibility and the guts, move foot to shoulder rest and go into a *Deep Split*—but use more resistance to stabilize the carriage

IMAGINE...*that your spine is growing taller every time you bring the carriage home.*

ELLIE SAYS...*"If you don't feel your inner thighs burning, move your feet farther apart or decrease resistance."*

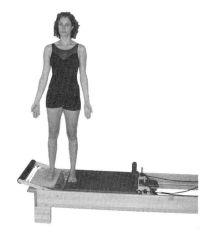

1. Starting Position—*8 to 10 repetitions*
Mount the machine without moving the carriage. Step first onto the footplate, then onto the carriage in either parallel or turn out. Spine and pelvis are neutral with hands on hips or down by sides.

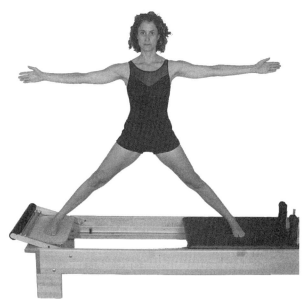

2. Inhale
Lengthen spine and press carriage away while raising arms to sides to shoulder height. Move carriage as far away from home as possible while maintaining Neutral Spine/Pelvis.

3. Exhale
Pull legs together to bring carriage home while lowering arms to sides.

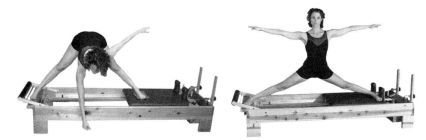

VARIATION: Pick a Flower   **ADVANCED VARIATION: Deep Split—Use more resistance!**

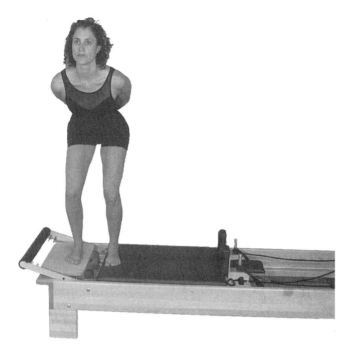

1. Starting Position—*8 repetitions*

Mount the machine without moving the carriage. Step first onto the foot plate, then onto the carriage. Legs in parallel, knees bent with torso pitched slightly forward and hands clasped behind pelvis (like a speed skater). Keep lumbar spine in neutral with abs pulling away from floor toward spine.

Inhale to prepare

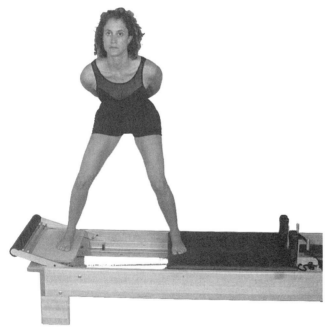

2. Exhale

Press carriage away, opening legs wider than shoulder distance, keeping pelvis centered between legs.

3. Inhale

Deepen abdominal engagement and pull legs together, bringing carriage home while keeping knees bent and weight evenly distributed between feet.

Repeat movement smoothly out and in.

MACHINE SET UP
- springs: 1 blue or 1 red
- bar: down with footplate installed
- ropes: N/A
- risers: N/A
- headrest: N/A

FUNCTIONS & TARGET MUSCLES
- Strengthens hip adductors and abductors
- Great for knee rehab

ALIGNMENT CUES & OBSTACLES
- Keep kneecaps forward and arches up and lifted
- Make sure big toe metatarsils stay in contact with footplate and carriage
- Keep back extended and navel lifted
- **Obstacles:** Tight Achilles tendon and tight plantar flexors

VARIATIONS & PEEL BACKS
- **Variation:** One leg at a time. Begin in *Bonnie Blair* Starting Position. Keep the leg on carriage stable as you press carriage out, straightening leg on footplate. Bend knee to come back home and repeat 5 times. Switch sides keeping leg on the footplate stable, and press carriage out by straightening leg on the carriage. Bring carriage home by bending leg on the carriage. Repeat 5 times

IMAGINE... *your knees are headlights shining straight forward as you go out and in.*

ELLIE SAYS... *"This is a great exercise for skiers, skaters, tennis players and anyone else who needs lateral stabilization of the knee."*

SPEED SKATING

MACHINE SET UP
- springs: 1 blue or 1 red
- bar: down with footplate installed
- ropes: N/A
- risers: N/A
- headrest: N/A

FUNCTIONS & TARGET MUSCLES
- Strengthens hip abductors and adductors
- Works ankle and knee stabilizers
- Mobilizes thoracic spine in rotation

ALIGNMENT CUES & OBSTACLES
- Keep movement fluid
- Keep head level throughout exercise (torso does not lower and rise)
- Rib cage rotates but pelvis remains square

IMAGINE... *you're skating for the gold.*

SUSI SAYS... *"I always feel more like an extra from the movie Xanadu than a speed skater when I do this exercise."*

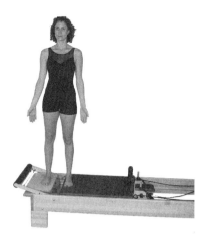

1. Starting Position—*8 to 10 repetitions*
Mount the machine without moving the carriage. Step first onto the footplate, then onto the carriage with parallel legs and arms relaxed by sides. Place feet as close to the edges as possible.

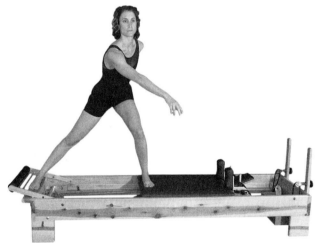

2. Exhale
Push carriage away from home with straight leg on footplate, bending leg on carriage. Pelvis shifts toward carriage leg.

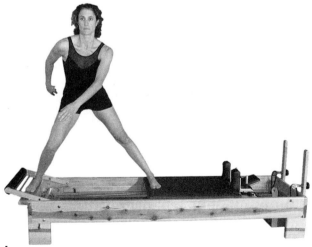

3. Inhale
Reverse the action, straightening leg on carriage and bending leg on footplate. Pelvis shifts toward footplate.

Repeat 2–3 times, then add spinal rotation toward bending knee and allow arms to follow torso movement. Arms should move in opposition to legs as a good skater would do.

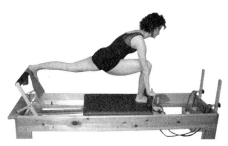

1. Starting Position—*3 to 5 preps, then 10 to 15 repetitions*

Facing back of Reformer, hold on to shoulder rests and place ball of right foot at the headrest crease, with knee bent to 90˚. Place left heel at corner of footbar with toes on metal arm. Inhale wide into back to prepare and press back heel into footbar.

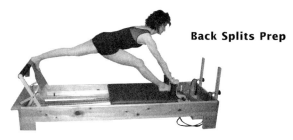

Back Splits Prep

2. Breathing Continuously

Maintain torso position, feeling abdominals pull to the spine, press back heel into bar, and straighten right knee, feeling VMO engage as you press heel into carriage. Do not hyperextend knee; keep hamstring engaged as you extend leg.

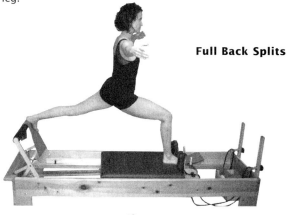

Full Back Splits

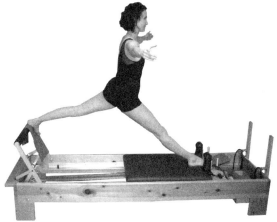

3. Breathing Continuously

From the bent knee position, keeping carriage and legs stable, bring torso upright, arms open to the sides. Press carriage out and in 10–15 times.

MACHINE SET UP

- springs: 1 red & 1 blue or yellow
- bar: high, with sticky pad on corner
- ropes: N/A
- risers: N/A
- headrest: up, with sticky pad

FUNCTIONS & TARGET MUSCLES

- Strengthens hamstrings, glutes and quads, especially VMO
- Advanced knee rehab
- Stretches hip flexors
- Challenges balance, control, and pelvic alignment
- Works abdominals, especially obliques, plus multifidi to prevent rotation of pelvis

ALIGNMENT CUES & OBSTACLES

- Keep pelvis as square as possible—focus on ASIS of extended leg staying front
- Keep bent knee tracking over second and third toe
- Press through big toe metatarsal of the moving leg to cue the VMO and hamstring
- Pelvis remains stationary in space—no up/down motion
- Really push the back heel into the bar to engage entire back of leg and glutes
- Do not snap front knee to straight—carriage should stay in motion until knee is fully extended (this prevents hyperextending the knee) and press heel into the carriage to keep hamstrings engaged
- Do not hyperextend lumbar spine—use abdominals to lift up pelvis
- Pelvis should never be lower than front knee
- Keep upper body relaxed and shoulders away from ears

VARIATIONS & PEEL BACKS

- **Modification:** Use low bar if client is very tall or has very tight hip flexors, but add spring resistance
- Use Pole at first for balance

IMAGINE...*your front knee is straightening from the back heel pressing into footbar.*

ELLIE SAYS...*"The front leg may be moving the carriage but the real work is in the back leg glutes."*

Use pole for balance

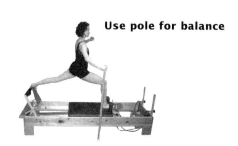

FRONT SPLITS: 4 PART STRETCH

MACHINE SET UP
- springs: 1 red & 1 blue or 1 yellow
- bar: high
- ropes: N/A
- risers: N/A
- headrest: N/A

FUNCTIONS & TARGET MUSCLES
- Stretches hip flexors and hamstrings
- Challenges balance
- Works your splits

ALIGNMENT CUES & OBSTACLES
- When stretching in the splits position, only extend as far as you can support the stretch
- For hamstring stretch, focus on back hip pulling forward to keep pelvis square
- Do not hyperextend knees or lock knees
- Do not hike a hip—keep both sides even
- Keep tension out of upper body while stretching legs

VARIATIONS & PEEL BACKS
- **Variation:** To deepen stretch on step 5, bring hands onto sides of Reformer
- **Peel Back:** *Psoas Stretch*

IMAGINE... *you're preparing for the Russian circus.*

ELLIE SAYS... *"Part Four is the best psoas stretch ever."*

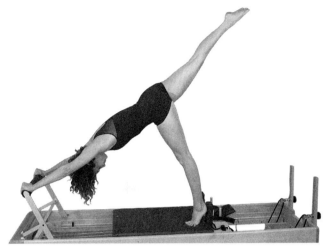

1. Starting Position—*1 repetition per side*
Start in *Arabesque* and allow carriage to move away from home.

Breathe continuously through this exercise, holding stretches for 3 to 4 breaths

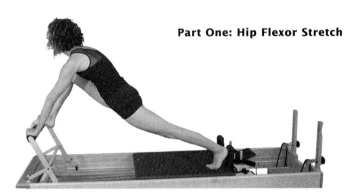

Part One: Hip Flexor Stretch

2. Breathing Continuously
Swing back leg forward, bending the knee and placing ball of foot on bar. Front knee is bent to 90° and back knee is straight, back heel against shoulder rest with toes forward. Hands are shoulder width apart on the bar. Push carriage away from home to stretch back leg hip flexors. Really press heel into shoulder rests to engage glutes and hamstrings. Keep front knee bent.

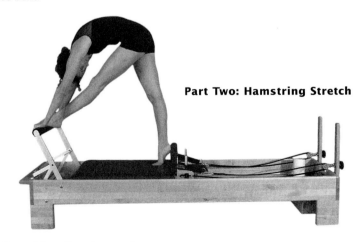

Part Two: Hamstring Stretch

3. Breathing Continuously
Bring carriage home as you straighten front knee to stretch hamstrings of front leg—keep pelvis square and don't jam front knee. Carriage should remain at home. Lift abdominals up to create a hovering feeling—don't drop down onto leg.

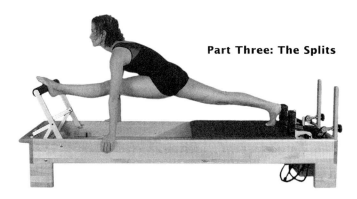

Part Three: The Splits

4. Breathing Continuously
Keep both knees straight and push carriage away from home, lowering pelvis between legs to come into splits position, keeping hips as square as possible. Keep abdominals engaged—don't sink into hips. (Grab onto the frame if you get down far enough.)

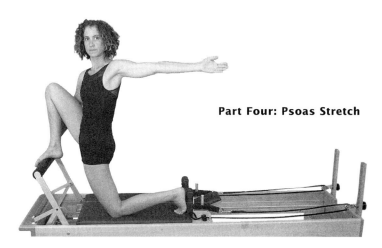

Part Four: Psoas Stretch

5. Breathing Continuously
Slowly lower back knee to carriage as front knee bends and carriage begins to move toward home. Bring torso upright and engage back glute to increase hip flexor stretch. Once carriage is home, raise one arm and circle it back, twisting ribcage—pelvis remains square to front. Reverse direction of circle and then switch sides.

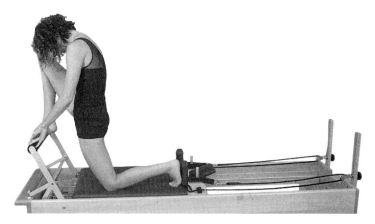

6. Dural Stretch
On inhale, lengthen spine then exhale and maintain length of spine while lowering chin to chest. Continue rounding spine down until you feel the "deep psoas" sensation—it should feel like you're actually stretching the lumbar attachment of the psoas (feel it in your back!).

MACHINE SET UP
- springs: 1 red & 1 blue or yellow
- bar: high
- ropes: N/A
- risers: N/A
- headrest: N/A

FUNCTIONS & TARGET MUSCLES
- Strengthens quads
- Challenges sense of balance
- Works abdominals, hamstrings, and glutes
- Stretches hip flexors and hamstrings

ALIGNMENT CUES & OBSTACLES
- Keep pelvis square as front knee straightens—no dipping or twisting
- Torso remains at same level in space while carriage moves—no bobbing up and down
- Spot by holding client's hand
- Keep hip, knee, and ankle in alignment
- Do not lock or hyperextend front knee while pushing carriage out—carriage should continue moving as knee straightens

VARIATIONS & PEEL BACKS
- Use a pole to assist and support client—this provides balance and greatly diminishes the "fear factor"
- **Peel Backs:** *Psoas Stretch, Front Splits: 4 Part Stretch*

IMAGINE...*you're painting the ceiling with your head—and if you don't remain level you will miss a spot (when doing bent leg variation).*

ELLIE SAYS...*"Use a pole if necessary."*

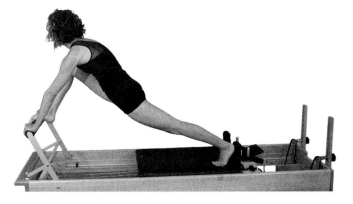

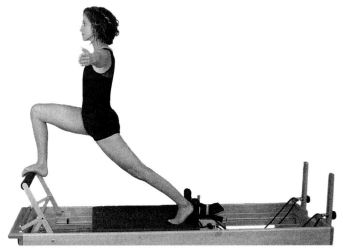

1. Starting Position—*4 to 8 repetitions on each side*
Lunge with ball of foot on bar and knee bent to 90°. Back leg is straight with foot in relevé position with heel pressing into shoulder rest. Hips are square. Then release hands from footbar and bring torso upright in one piece, opening arms out to sides (2nd position). If using a pole, hand it to client once they are upright.

Inhale and lengthen spine to prepare

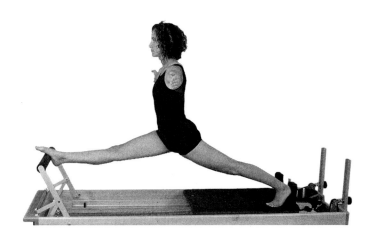

2. Exhale
Pull abdominals to spine to maintain length in torso, and push carriage away from home by straightening front knee. Think of pressing back and forward, not up and down. You should not loose any height in your head.

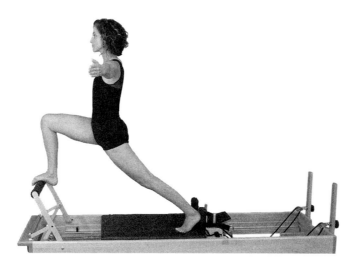

3. Inhale
Bend front knee and return to Starting Position while lengthening spine.

Repeat 4 to 8 times. With carriage home, transition into straight leg version by straightening front leg without moving the carriage.

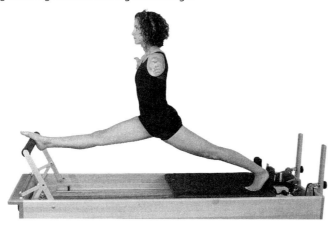

4. Exhale
Pull abdominals to spine and move carriage away from home lowering pelvis between legs. Keep the ASIS of back leg pointed forward as hip goes further and further into extension.

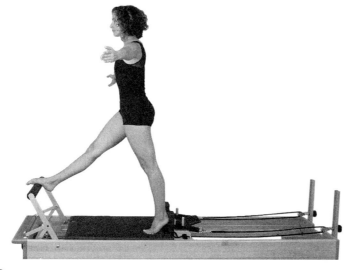

5. Inhale
Focus on drawing inner thighs together while controlling carriage back to home and lengthening spine out of pelvis. Torso/head do not remain level in this variation.

JUMPING PREP/FOOTWORK

MACHINE SET UP
- springs: 2 reds & 1 blue
- bar: behind jumpboard for stability
- headrest: up

FUNCTIONS & TARGET MUSCLES
- Teaches articulation through the foot and proper landing from the jump

ALIGNMENT CUES & OBSTACLES
- Think: bend, straight, toes then heels, bend, straight, toes then heels
- Only bend your knees as far as you can keep your heels in contact with the jumpboard

VARIATIONS & PEEL BACKS
- **Footwork on the Jumpboard:** (not shown) *Footwork on the Jumpboard.* A great warm-up for jumping as well as a fantastic functional challenge! Use the same props as you would for parallel footwork on the Footbar

  In Parallel with Feet Planted: Start with feet toward the top of the Jumpboard, hip distance apart, and keep "all four tires" of feet in contact with Jumpboard, focusing on knees aligning over middle of foot, heels grounded as you bend in. This exercise is excellent for strengthening the ankle and correcting pronation/supination patterns. This is the most functional Footwork position, and translates directly to gait

  Parallel on Toes: Keep weight distributed equally through the base of the metatarsal, particularly the big toe metatarsal, and keep heels lifted and aligned with the center of the metatarsal base

  Parallel Combo: Start on toes and straighten legs out, then roll down to heels so the whole foot is planted, then bend in as far as you can keeping heels grounded, and slowly roll back up to the toes. Repeat 5 times and reverse. Great for stretching and strengthening the feet and ankles, and training articulation of foot for landing in Jumping

  First Position with Feet Planted: Same as Parallel with Feet Planted, but turned out

  First Position on Toes: Feet turned out with heels together and lifted

  First Position Combo: Same as Parallel Combo, but turned out with heels staying together the whole time (adjust feet as necessary to make this happen)

  Second Position: Wide turned-out position with heels on the edges of jumpboard—toes off the edge

IMAGINE...*you are doing pliés in ballet class.*

ELLIE SAYS...*"Non-dancers need to learn how to use their feet properly when they jump!"*

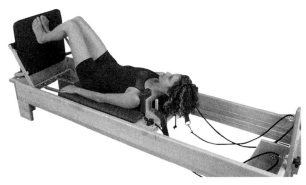

1. Starting Position—*8 repetitions*
Lie on the carriage with legs together in parallel, knees bent with feet flat, placed toward the top of the jumpboard.

Inhale to prepare

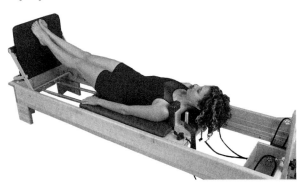

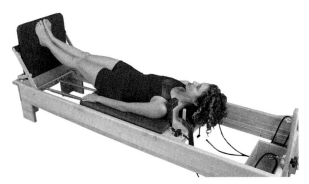

2. Exhale
Straighten the legs, then rise up onto your toes, then come back down to flat feet.

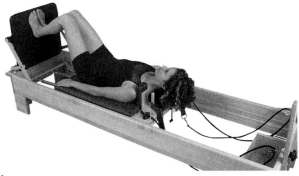

3. Exhale
Bend your knees back to the Starting Position.

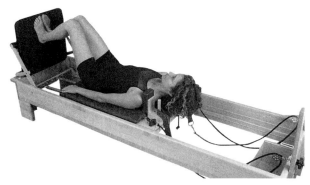

1. Starting Position—*8 to 16 jumps in parallel*
Lie on the carriage with legs together in parallel, knees bent with feet flat, placed toward the top of the jumpboard.

Inhale to prepare

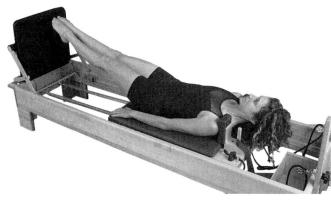

2. Exhale
Straighten the legs and jump, pointing your toes in the air.

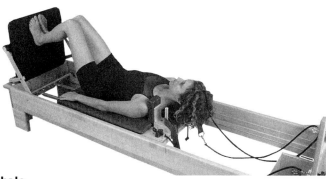

3. Inhale
Land like a cat, making no noise at all, articulating through your feet and bending your knees back to the Starting Position. Do not let heels come off jumpboard when landing!

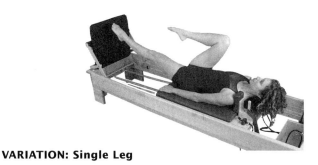

VARIATION: Single Leg

MACHINE SET UP
- springs: 2 reds
- bar: high, with jumpboard installed into slot. Loosen the knobs on the front of the Reformer to loosen the metal jumpboard slot. Place the wooden insert into the slot and slide the footbar up and over the wooden slat on the back of the jumpboard (this is what stabilizes the jumpboard). Finally, tighten the front knobs
- headrest: up

FUNCTIONS & TARGET MUSCLES
- Teaches articulation through the foot and proper landing from the jump.
- Strengthens lower limb in explosive movement
- Great for advanced rehab of foot, knee, ankle and hip
- Aerobic challenge

ALIGNMENT CUES & OBSTACLES
- Feet should be pointed in the air—no flaccid feet!
- Only bend your knees as far as you can keep your heels in contact with the jumpboard
- Press your heels into the jumpboard to try to engage your hamstrings as much as possible

VARIATIONS & PEEL BACKS
- **Variation:** Try *Jumping* in turn out, allowing the legs to open slightly in midair
- **Variation:** *Single Leg Jumping* (in parallel or turn out)
- **Variation:** Try *Jumping Combo* (in parallel or turn out) for an aerobic challenge:
  - 8 jumps with both legs/ 8 jumps on right leg/ 8 jumps on the left leg
  - 4 jumps with both legs/ 4 jumps on right leg/ 4 jumps on the left leg
  - 2 jumps with both legs/ 2 jumps on right leg/ 2 jumps on the left leg
  - 1 jump with both legs/ 1 jump on right leg/ 1 jump on the left leg/ repeat the 1's
- **Peel Back:** *Jumping Prep*

IMAGINE...*you are doing jumps in ballet class.*

ELLIE SAYS...*"Don't be afraid to have your injured clients do this exercise before they return to dancing, running or any other impact activity."*

super advanced repertoire

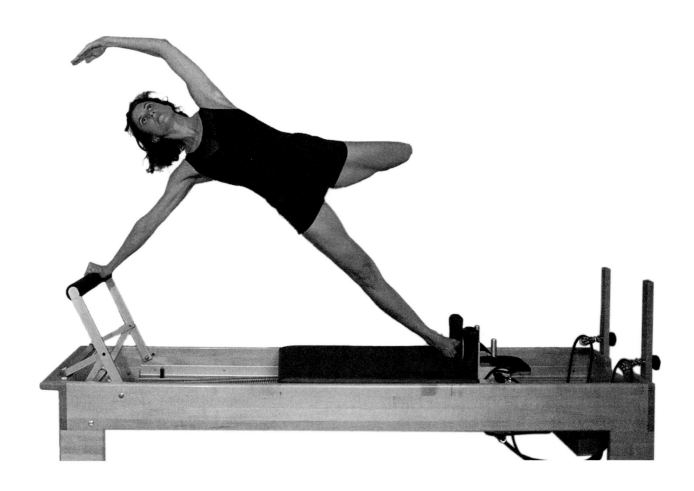

The following exercises are some of the most challenging in the repertoire. They all require a great deal of core strength, and certain ones really challenge the upper body. Reserve these for your advanced clients who want to be pushed to their ultimate limits. They are great for precision athletes like dancers, gymnasts, circus performers, etc. If they seem impossible at first, come back when you're stronger and try them again. Don't forget about them!

SUPER ADVANCED EXERCISES
Thread The Needle/Star Prep
Star
Snake
Twist
Corkscrew
Control Balance Dismount
Backbend

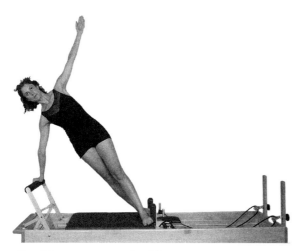

MACHINE SET UP
- springs: 1 red & 1 blue or 1 yellow
- bar: high
- ropes: N/A
- risers: N/A
- headrest: N/A

FUNCTIONS & TARGET MUSCLES
- Challenges stability of core and shoulder
- Works lats, abdominals, hip flexors and glutes

ALIGNMENT CUES & OBSTACLES
- Make sure not to arch low back when opening the chest—think of your sternum turning to the sky while your ASIS's shine forward like headlights, stretching your chest without taxing your low back
- Keep hips lifted away from the carriage when pushing away from home
- Focus on shoulder stability, feeling scapulae reach towards pelvis
- **Contraindications:** Wrist and/or shoulder issues, disc dysfunction, osteoporosis

VARIATIONS & PEEL BACKS
- **Peel Back:** *Advanced Mermaid/Side Plank on the Mat*

IMAGINE...*you are Threading a Needle—which is you!*

ELLIE SAYS...*"This exercise is much less scary than the Star and it's a great way to prep for it."*

1. Starting Position—*once each side*
Stand at side of Reformer and place hand in center of footbar. Place the inside of foot that is closest to the footbar against the closest shoulder rest. Place the outside of the second foot against the far shoulder rest. With top leg forward and your bottom leg back, reach your free arm up to the sky.

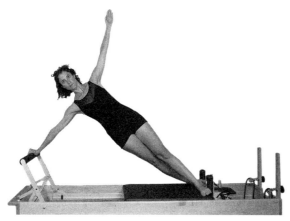

2. Inhale
Press the carriage away from home as far as you can without losing shoulder stability.

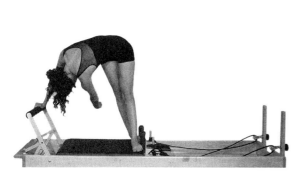

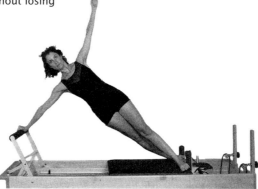

3. Exhale
Bring the carriage home by folding your body in half, scooping abdominals, then *Thread the Needle* by bringing your free arm through the arc of your body, reaching it behind you as you twist towards the floor.

4. Inhale
Unfold your body as you press the carriage out, reaching your arm back up, this time opening your chest to sky at the farthest point, allowing your arm to reach slightly backward, keeping the hips square and pointing forward.

Repeat Step 2–3 four times and then dismount and change sides.

STAR

MACHINE SET UP
- springs: 1 red & 1 blue or yellow
- bar: high
- ropes: N/A
- risers: N/A
- headrest: N/A

FUNCTIONS & TARGET MUSCLES
- Challenges core and shoulder stability
- Works lats, abdominals, hip flexors and glutes

ALIGNMENT CUES & OBSTACLES
- This is a *Star*, not a *Side Plank*, so don't let your hips drop, keep them lifted toward the sky—this will give you a feeling of lightness on your supporting arm
- Do not hyperextend lumbar spine when reaching leg into extension—keep movement at the hip joint
- **Contraindications:** Wrist and/or shoulder issues

VARIATIONS & PEEL BACKS
- **Peel Backs:** *Thread the Needle* on the Reformer, the *Star* on the Mat, and *Side Kicks* on PhysioBall

IMAGINE...*your free arm is an unmoving pole of support as carriage moves in and out and leg moves forward and back.*

ELLIE SAYS...*"This is the one exercise all the students get scared to perform on their final practical exam. But it's really not that bad!"*

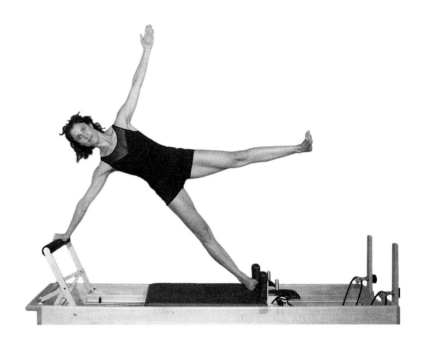

1. Starting Position—*once each side*
Stand at side of Reformer and place hand in center of footbar. Place the inside of foot that is closest to the footbar against the closest shoulder rest. Lift up into your *Star* position, with the hips lifting up to the sky and top leg reaching diagonally up to the sky. Carriage will move away from home as you assume the *Star* position. After mounting, reach free arm forward so that it is parallel to floor in Door Frame position.

Inhale to prepare

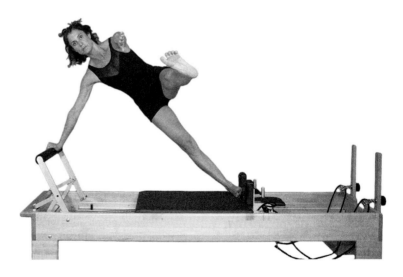

2. Exhale
Kick the top leg forward toward hand as the carriage moves closer to home. Foot of top leg is flexed. Torso stays long and aligned.

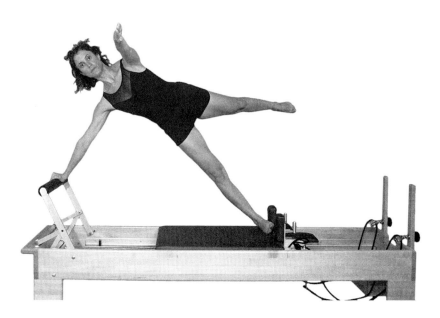

3. Inhale

Allow carriage to move away from home as you extend the top leg behind you, keeping knee straight and pointing the foot. Keep top arm stationary and energized, as in an arabesque. Keep pelvis lifted and square.

Repeat kicks front and back 3 times.

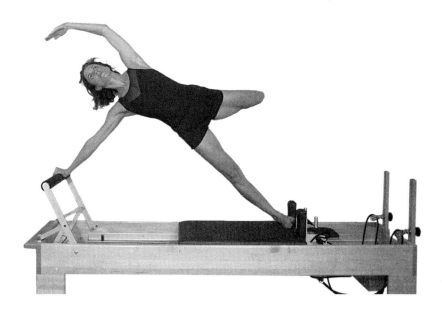

4. Exhale

On the 3rd arabesque, come into a back "attitude" by bending knee of top leg as it reaches behind you. Raise free arm and reach it overhead. Begin the dismount by bringing the back leg down to the floor behind you, controlling the carriage back home.

SNAKE

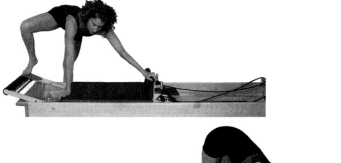

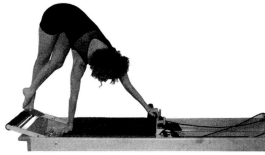

MACHINE SET UP

- springs: 1 red or blue & 1 yellow
- bar: down, with sticky pad on the close corner
- ropes: N/A
- risers: N/A
- headrest: N/A

FUNCTIONS & TARGET MUSCLES

- Strengthens the lats, back extensors, arms, quads, and core
- Teaches sequencing of the spine
- Peel back for the *Twist*

ALIGNMENT CUES & OBSTACLES

- Keep hips square with shoulders
- Keep the non-weight-bearing leg soft at the knee
- Keep the belly lifted and really scooped, and the shoulders down away from the ears when you are out in your full back extension
- **Obstacles:** weak upper back, tight hamstrings
- **Contraindications:** Wrist and/or shoulder issues, disc dysfunction, osteoporosis and stenosis

VARIATIONS & PEEL BACKS

- **Modification:** If your lats aren't strong enough to support your body weight, try placing your far hand down on the carriage instead of on top of the shoulder rest
- **Peel Back:** *Around the World/Up Stretch*

IMAGINE... Think Snake!

ELLIE SAYS...*"This exercise is a lot like Around the World/Up Stretch, but we're adding asymmetry to the mix."*

1. Starting Position—*3 repetitions*
Stand on the side of the Reformer and place one hand on top of the far shoulder rest, fingers facing the risers, and place the other hand on the bottom edge of the carriage, fingers wrapped around the edge. Then mount the Reformer by placing your near foot onto a sticky pad covering the corner of the footbar, lift your body up lightly from the center, fold in half and, without moving the carriage, lift the heel of the standing leg up to a relevé, and cross your free foot in front of the standing foot, so that there is no weight-bearing by the front leg. Square your hips with your shoulders.

Inhale to prepare

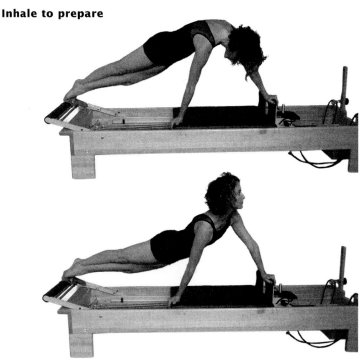

2. Exhale
Press the carriage out, keeping your hips square to the shoulders so that the hip bones aim straight down to the carriage. *Snake* your spine slowly into extension by tucking your pelvis under, squeezing your glutes and lifting from your belly. Then slowly ripple your spine into extension from the base to the top: lower back, upper back, neck and head.

3. Inhale
Return home by un-snaking the spine, sequencing the flexion from bottom to top, starting by again tucking the pelvis, then belly scooping the belly to lift the lower back, upper back, neck and head.

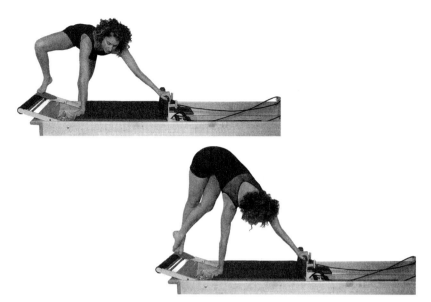

1. Starting Position—*3 repetitions*

Stand on the side of the Reformer and place one hand on top of the far shoulder rest, fingers facing the risers, and place the other hand on the bottom edge of the carriage, fingers wrapped around the edge. Then mount the Reformer by placing your near foot onto a sticky pad covering the corner of the footbar, lift your body up lightly from the center, fold in half, and, without moving the carriage, lift the heel of the standing leg up to a relevé, and cross your free foot in front of the standing foot, with only the toes down so that there is no weight-bearing by the front leg. Square your hips with your shoulders.

Inhale to prepare

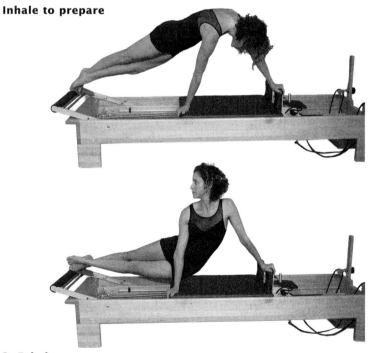

2. Exhale

Press the carriage out as you do in the *Snake*, leading with your pelvis tucking under. Stop the carriage halfway and allow your hips to rotate and drop down toward the carriage as the heel of your supporting foot comes down onto the footbar to ground you. Finish by turning your head in the direction of your toes.

3. Inhale

Return home by untwisting and lifting your pelvis so that the hip bones are once again square with the shoulders, allowing the heel of the supporting foot to lift into relevé, and fold back in half.

MACHINE SET UP

- springs: 1 red or blue & 1 yellow
- bar: down, with sticky pad on the close corner
- ropes: N/A
- risers: N/A
- headrest: N/A

FUNCTIONS & TARGET MUSCLES

- Strengthens the lats, back extensors, arms, quads, and core
- Deeply stretches the quadratus lumborum and abdominal obliques

ALIGNMENT CUES & OBSTACLES

- Press into the arms to engage the lats and to lift the body weight away from gravity
- Keep the non-weight-bearing knee soft
- It is very important to allow the foot of the supporting leg to go from relevé to flat on the footbar during the twisting movement—this allows the supporting leg to rotate at the same time that the pelvis does, so that the knee does not torque in the process
- **Obstacles:** Weak upper body, especially lats
- **Contraindications:** Wrist and/or shoulder issues, disc dysfunction, osteoporosis, stenosis

VARIATIONS & PEEL BACKS

- **Modification:** If your lats aren't strong enough to support your body weight, try placing your far hand on the carriage instead of on top of the shoulder rest
- **Peel Back:** *Snake*

IMAGINE...*someday this won't seem so hard.*

ELLIE SAYS...*"When I first learned Twist years ago, I thought that it was ridiculously hard and what's the point? Now that I have enough lat strength to do it right, I think it's the best QL stretch ever."*

CORKSCREW

MACHINE SET UP
- springs: all
- bar: down
- ropes: N/A
- risers: N/A
- headrest: down

FUNCTIONS & TARGET MUSCLES
- Stretches and articulates the spine
- Strengthens the hip flexors, inner thighs and abdominals, especially the abdominal obliques

ALIGNMENT CUES & OBSTACLES
- Make sure to reach your tailbone long away from you as you roll down your spine—don't let the hips hike toward your head
- Try to keep the elbows wide and the shoulders down the back
- **Contraindications:** disc dysfunction, osteoporosis, neck sensitivity/injury

VARIATIONS & PEEL BACKS
- **Advanced Variation:** *Corkscrew Around the World*: Make one huge circle with your legs, keeping your hips in Levitation as you descend and ascend
- **Peel Backs:** *Overhead, Corkscrew* on the Mat

IMAGINE...*you are doing an Overhead with a Twist.*

ELLIE SAYS...*"The Corkscrew is a counter-intuitive movement—watch the direction of the legs as you twist your hips (the direction in which they fall is the first half of the circle). Think of making a G clef shape with your legs—not a circle!"*

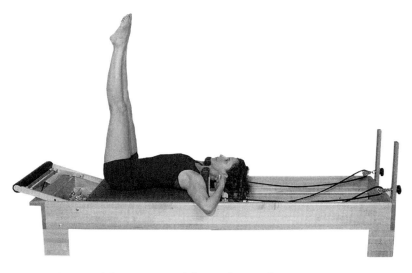

1. Starting Position—*4 repetitions alternating*
Lie on your back on the carriage, holding onto the pegs, elbows wide, and legs in Pilates First Position, reaching straight up to the sky. Make sure to keep your belly pulled in and your back flat on the carriage.

Inhale to prepare

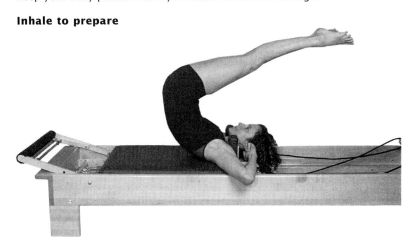

2. Inhale
Lift your legs up and over your head.

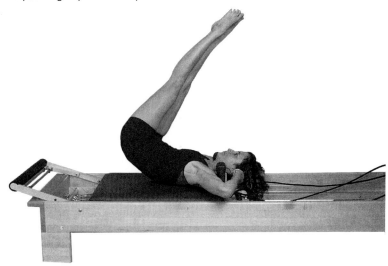

3. Exhale
Twist your hips to the right, and articulate down the right side of your spine, along the spinal erectors, with your tailbone reaching straight down toward the footbar, and your legs at an angle toward the right.

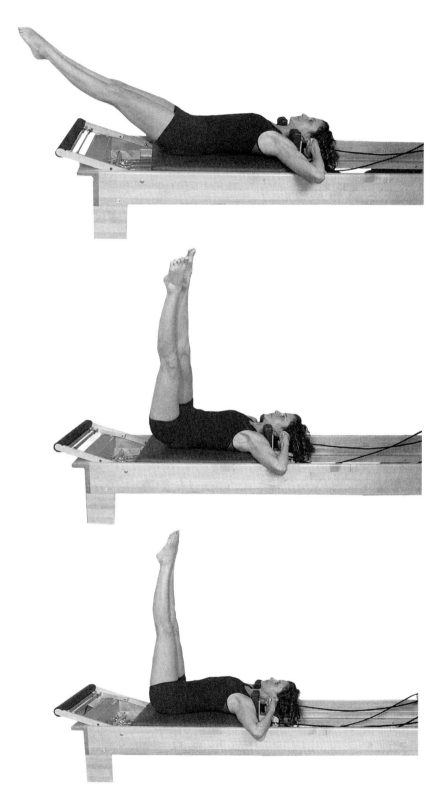

4. Inhale
Once your tail has landed, complete the circle of the legs by bringing them down, to the left, and to the center.

Exhale and reverse directions.

CONTROL BALANCE DISMOUNT

MACHINE SET UP
- springs: all
- bar: down
- ropes: N/A
- risers: N/A
- head rest: down

FUNCTIONS & TARGET MUSCLES
- Challenges balance, control, strength, and flexibility
- Works glutes, abdominals, pecs, and deltoids
- Impresses your friends, and is not as hard as it looks

ALIGNMENT CUES & OBSTACLES
- Really reach top leg to the ceiling as you dismount—this is the trick of the exercise!
- Keep shoulders wide with elbows out to the sides and weight balanced between shoulder blades
- Lower the leg as close to the frame as possible—especially when you're going to stand on it
- When remounting onto Reformer, aim your head lower than the headrest
- How are you going to stay out of your neck? By pushing off the Reformer with your arm strength, and of course by using the abdominals and glutes
- Use opposing energy between top and bottom legs to keep body light
- The leg pointed to the ceiling is the arabesque leg and never touches the floor
- **Obstacles:** Weak core, inflexible spine, poor sense of balance, tight hamstrings
- **Contraindications:** Neck injuries, disc dysfunction, osteoporosis

VARIATIONS & PEEL BACKS
- **Variation:** (for extra credit) In step 6, maintain Levitation in hips as you switch sides
- **Peel Backs:** Practice backwards-over-the-shoulder somersaults on Mat, *Control Balance* on the Mat

IMAGINE...*you are being lifted off the carriage by the hand of the Pilates Goddess grabbing onto your ankle and levitating you up to the sky.*

ELLIE SAYS... *"Control Balance Dismount is crazy...crazy fun!"*

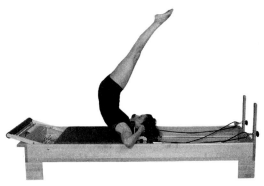

1. Starting Position—*one rep on each side*
Lying supine on carriage with hips flexed to 90° and in slight external rotation, making Pilates "V". Hold pegs keeping elbows wide and Levitate up into shoulder stand—keeping weight on upper back. Knees are straight and toes are pointed.

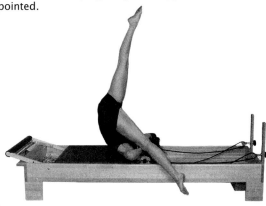

2. Inhale
Lower one leg down with foot coming to the outside of Reformer, as the top leg reaches up to the sky, splitting the legs in counter stretch.

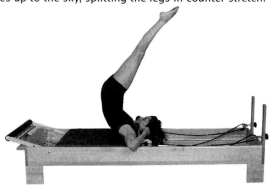

3. Exhale
Raise leg back to line of body. Lower and raise the leg twice more.

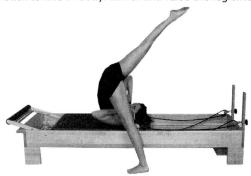

4. Breathing Continuously
Lower the leg, bend at waist, bring foot down to floor close to Reformer, and begin to roll over shoulder. Top leg continues to reach up. Using arms and abdominals, continue to roll over shoulder (like a back somersault), peeling torso off machine and end in an arabesque standing next to Reformer. Use arms to help you push body off machine.

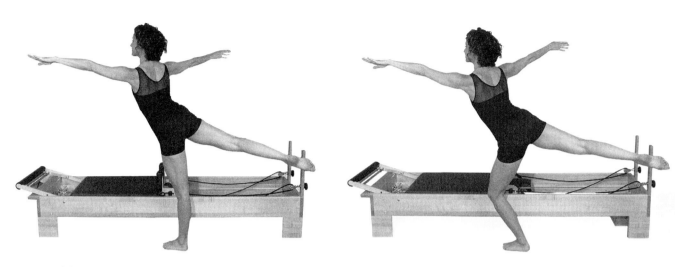

5. Breathing Continuously

Open both arms out to the sides (2nd position), and maintain height and arabesque shape of back leg while bending the standing knee (plié). Straighten knee and rise onto toes (relevé). Keep the abdominals up and lifted to improve balance.

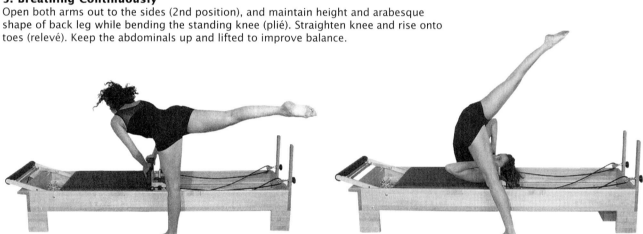

6. Breathing Continuously

Keeping back leg straight and energized, somersault back onto Reformer holding pegs and aiming head onto carriage. Abdominals remain engaged to control momentum. Tuck head into headrest and put body weight on upper back—not neck! Levitate lifted leg up to sky to lighten the load.

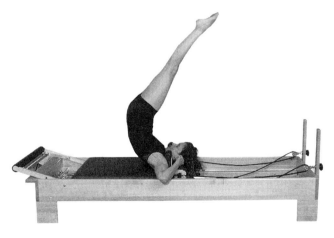

7. Breathing Continuously

Levitate legs up to the sky in shoulder stand and alternate sides.

To finish from shoulder stand roll down sequentially through spine.

BACKBEND

MACHINE SET UP

- springs: 3 red springs
- bar: down, with sticky pads on the corners
- ropes: N/A
- risers: N/A
- headrest: up or down

FUNCTIONS & TARGET MUSCLES

- Stretches the abdominals, hip flexors, chest, lats, and pecs
- Strengthens the glutes, lower back, shoulders, and arms

ALIGNMENT CUES & OBSTACLES

- Make sure to keep the lower body stable so that the fulcrum of the pulsing emanates from the chest and shoulders not the lower back
- Use your glutes to help decompress the low back
- **Contraindications:** SI joint instability, stenosis, shoulder and/or wrist problems

VARIATIONS & PEEL BACKS

- **Peel Back:** Try a *Backbend* on the floor first

IMAGINE...*your sternum is breaking open as you bring the carriage in.*

ELLIE SAYS...*"This is another part of the Pilates X files."*

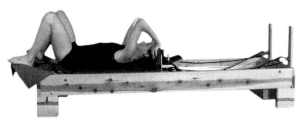

1. Starting Position—*one repetition with 8 slow pulses*
Start lying supine on the carriage with your head on the head rest and then place your feet on the corners of the footbar, slightly externally rotated so that the feet feel secure on the sticky pads. Reach your arms up to the sky and them bend them so that the elbows stick straight up and the palms come down on the shoulder rests, fingers pointing toward the toes.

Inhale to prepare

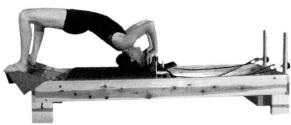

2. Exhale
Press into your arms and feet and come up to a half-backbend first, resting the top of your head on the head rest. Then straighten the arms all the way to a full backbend. The carriage should not move very much.

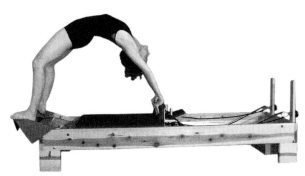

3. Inhale
Press the carriage out with your arms, keeping the lower body stable.

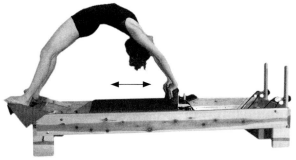

4. Exhale
Allow the chest to open as you bring the carriage back in. This is a deep lat stretch, so think of the stretch axis at the armpit, not the spine.

Repeat the arm movements 8 times, then retrograde coming back down, first stopping in the half-backbend position.

reformer exercise index

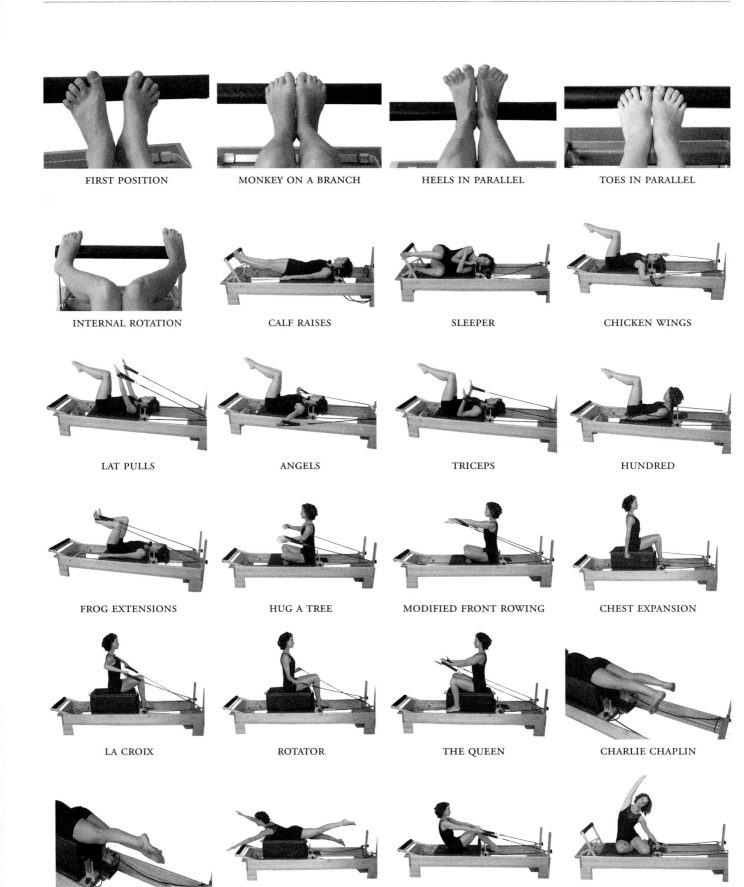

FIRST POSITION MONKEY ON A BRANCH HEELS IN PARALLEL TOES IN PARALLEL

INTERNAL ROTATION CALF RAISES SLEEPER CHICKEN WINGS

LAT PULLS ANGELS TRICEPS HUNDRED

FROG EXTENSIONS HUG A TREE MODIFIED FRONT ROWING CHEST EXPANSION

LA CROIX ROTATOR THE QUEEN CHARLIE CHAPLIN

SCISSORS SWIMMING ROLL DOWNS MERMAID

beginning series continued

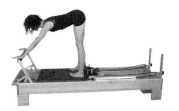

ELEPHANT: FLAT BACK

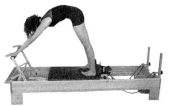

ELEPHANT: ROUND BACK

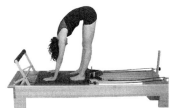

FORWARD BEND STRETCH

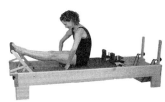

STOMACH MASSAGE: ROUND BACK

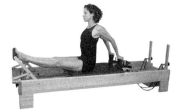

STOMACH MASSAGE: FLAT BACK

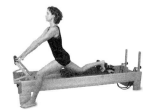

PSOAS STRETCH

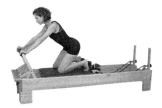

KNEE STRETCH: FLAT BACK

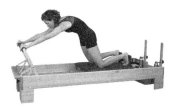

KNEE STRETCH: ROUND BACK

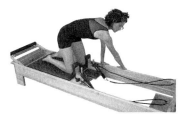

REVERSE KNEE STRETCH SERIES

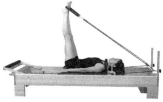

LEG PULLS IN PARALLEL

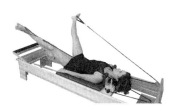

OPEN & CLOSE

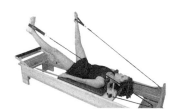

OPEN & CLOSE: TURN OUT & IN

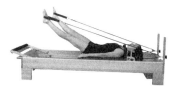

RECTANGLES

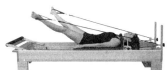

CIRCLES: TURN OUT

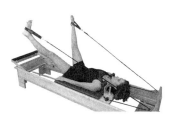

OVALS: TURN IN

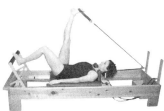

3 WAY HIP STRETCH: HAMSTRINGS

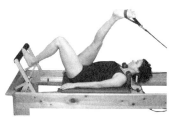

3 WAY HIP STRETCH: ITB

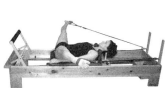

3 WAY HIP STRETCH: ADDUCTORS

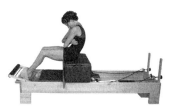

ROUND BACK ROLL DOWN

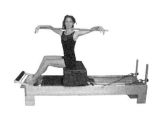

OLD MAN AT THE GYM

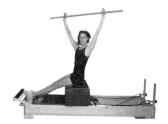

TWIST WITH A STICK

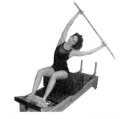

UP & OVER A BARREL

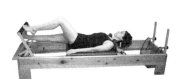

PRANCING

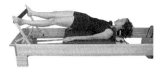

BOTTOM LIFT

intermediate series

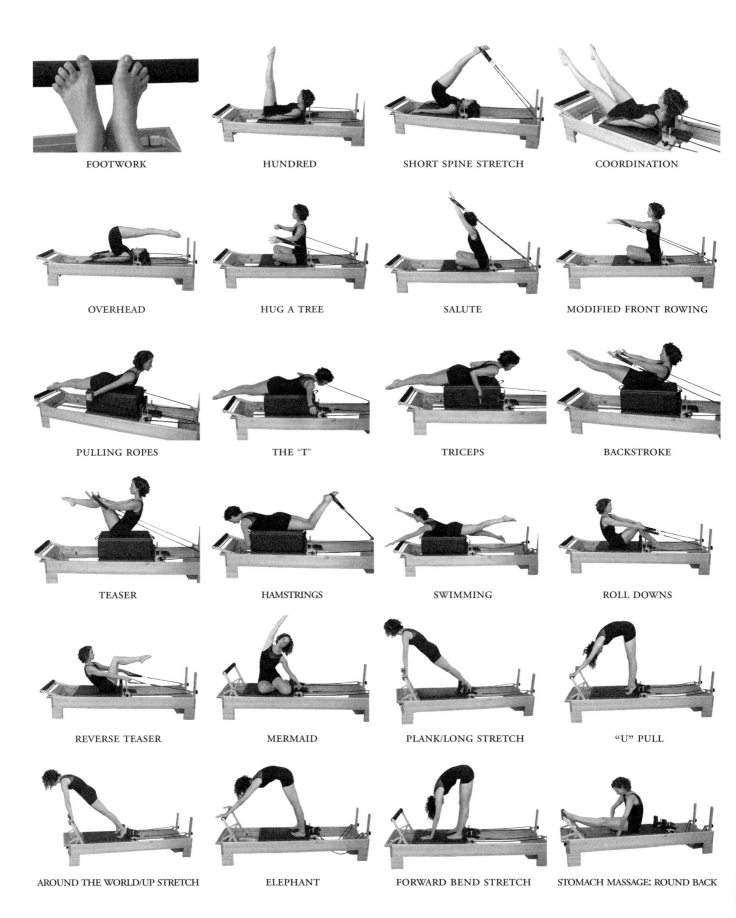

FOOTWORK

HUNDRED

SHORT SPINE STRETCH

COORDINATION

OVERHEAD

HUG A TREE

SALUTE

MODIFIED FRONT ROWING

PULLING ROPES

THE "T"

TRICEPS

BACKSTROKE

TEASER

HAMSTRINGS

SWIMMING

ROLL DOWNS

REVERSE TEASER

MERMAID

PLANK/LONG STRETCH

"U" PULL

AROUND THE WORLD/UP STRETCH

ELEPHANT

FORWARD BEND STRETCH

STOMACH MASSAGE: ROUND BACK

intermediate series continued

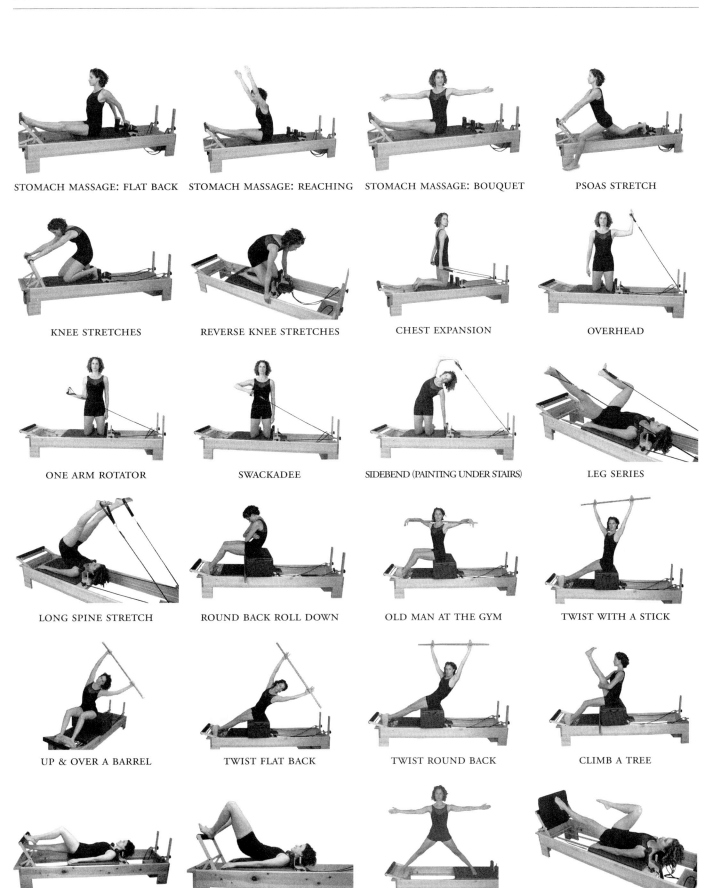

STOMACH MASSAGE: FLAT BACK STOMACH MASSAGE: REACHING STOMACH MASSAGE: BOUQUET PSOAS STRETCH

KNEE STRETCHES REVERSE KNEE STRETCHES CHEST EXPANSION OVERHEAD

ONE ARM ROTATOR SWACKADEE SIDEBEND (PAINTING UNDER STAIRS) LEG SERIES

LONG SPINE STRETCH ROUND BACK ROLL DOWN OLD MAN AT THE GYM TWIST WITH A STICK

UP & OVER A BARREL TWIST FLAT BACK TWIST ROUND BACK CLIMB A TREE

PRANCING BOTTOM LIFT SIDE SPLIT SERIES JUMPING

advanced series

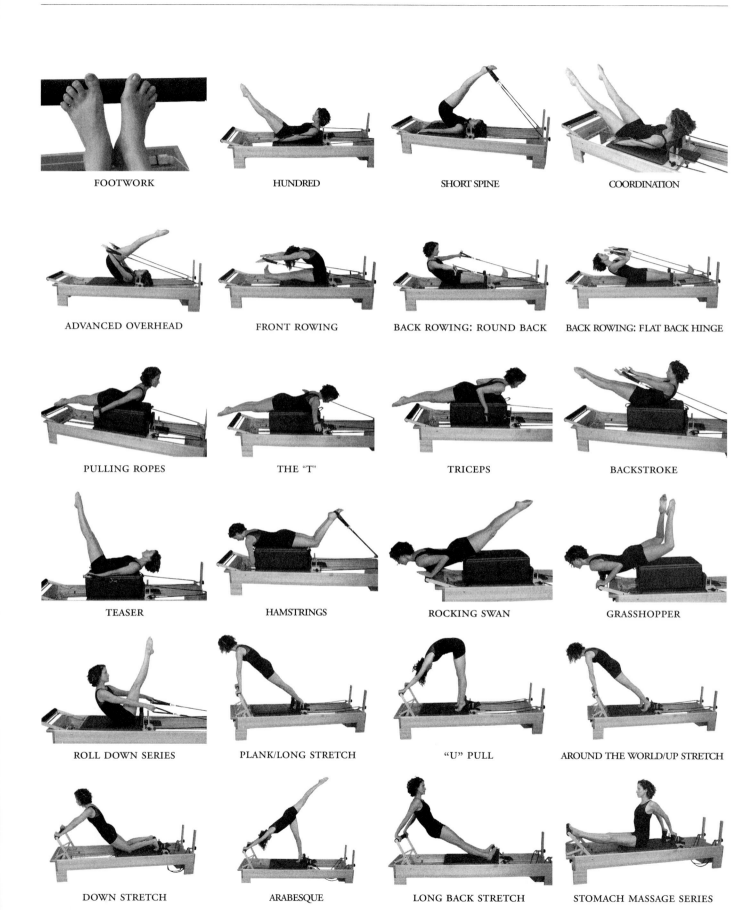

FOOTWORK

HUNDRED

SHORT SPINE

COORDINATION

ADVANCED OVERHEAD

FRONT ROWING

BACK ROWING: ROUND BACK

BACK ROWING: FLAT BACK HINGE

PULLING ROPES

THE "T"

TRICEPS

BACKSTROKE

TEASER

HAMSTRINGS

ROCKING SWAN

GRASSHOPPER

ROLL DOWN SERIES

PLANK/LONG STRETCH

"U" PULL

AROUND THE WORLD/UP STRETCH

DOWN STRETCH

ARABESQUE

LONG BACK STRETCH

STOMACH MASSAGE SERIES

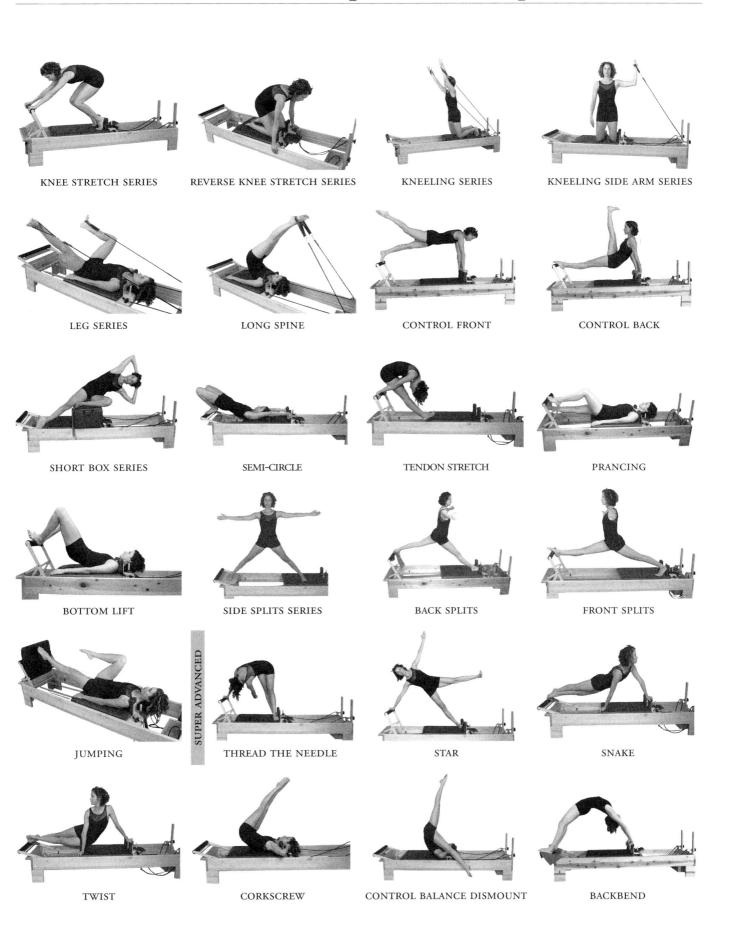

KNEE STRETCH SERIES

REVERSE KNEE STRETCH SERIES

KNEELING SERIES

KNEELING SIDE ARM SERIES

LEG SERIES

LONG SPINE

CONTROL FRONT

CONTROL BACK

SHORT BOX SERIES

SEMI-CIRCLE

TENDON STRETCH

PRANCING

BOTTOM LIFT

SIDE SPLITS SERIES

BACK SPLITS

FRONT SPLITS

JUMPING

SUPER ADVANCED

THREAD THE NEEDLE

STAR

SNAKE

TWIST

CORKSCREW

CONTROL BALANCE DISMOUNT

BACKBEND

OTHER BOOKS BY ELLIE HERMAN

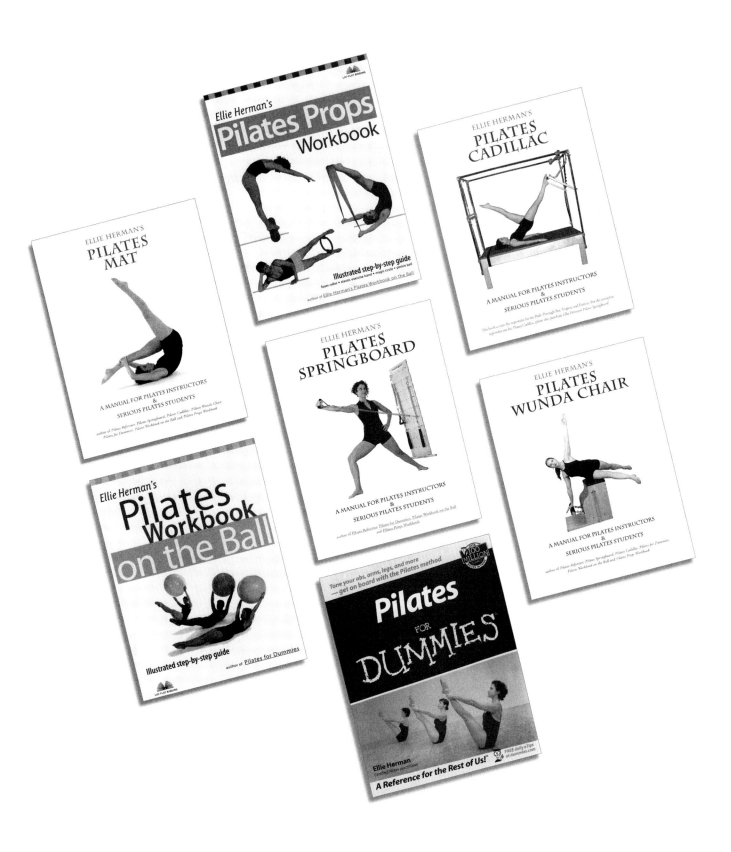

THE PILATES SPRINGBOARD
DESIGNED BY ELLIE HERMAN

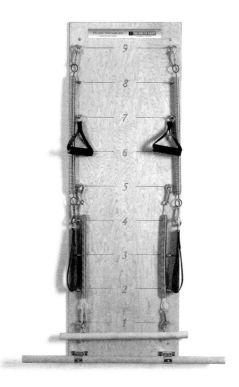

The Pilates Springboard is a space saving and affordable piece of resistance equipment which gives you a full-body workout. The Pilates Springboard consists of a 5-foot rectangular wooden board with eyelets placed on either side at 6" increments and a dowel at the bottom to use for arm or foot support. It comes with:

• two arm springs with neoprene handles

• two leg springs, with cotton loops

• one wooden roll-back bar

The Pilates Springboard comes with a 45 minute flow workout video which takes you through a warm-up, core strengthening, upper body and lower body conditioning program. Some of the exercises are from classic Pilates repertoire, and others are original exercises developed by master Pilates teacher Ellie Herman especially for the Springboard.

The Pilates Springboard is bolted into studs for support, taking up no floor space. This makes it perfect for an extra room, a home gym, garage, attic, or basement. For those with gyms or Pilates studios, you can affordably mount several Springboards along a wall and offer challenging Pilates group equipment classes without moving heavy equipment or taking up valuable storage space.

The Pilates Springboard costs $395
plus tax and shipping, and includes an instructional video.
Manufactured by **Balanced Body**, the leader in Pilates equipment.

Ellie Herman Studios distributes **Balanced Body** Equipment. Buy a Springboard or any piece of
Balanced Body Equipment and receive 5% of your purchase price
in products or services at any of our locations.

Pilates Springboard classes offered everyday at our studios—come check them out!

ELLIE HERMAN STUDIO SELLS MBT SHOES

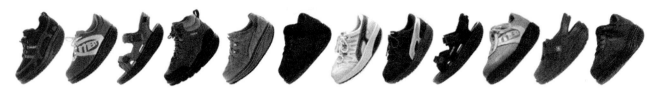

Masai Barefoot Technology—It's like doing Pilates while you walk.

Gentle, active rolling instead of repeated compression leads to relaxed, natural standing and walking.

• facilitates optimal posture and gait

• significantly reduces joint compression (spine, hips and knees)

• corrects imbalances and compensations

• tones your legs, hips and buns

• increases circulation

• rehabilitates spine, hip, knee, and ankle injuries

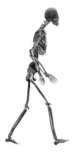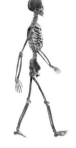

WITHOUT MBT   WITH MBT

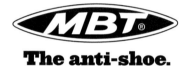

The anti-shoe.

MBT + PILATES = WALK-ILATES℠

Walk-ilates was developed by master Pilates teacher Ellie Herman to maximize the MBT walking experience. The class begins with special releases and stretches using the ethafoam roller, followed by Pilates Mat exercises and standing balances using the Magic Circle (all done in your MBTs). The class culminates in walking outside where proper gait and optimal alignment are stressed. Everyone will receive personal corrections to address their gait patterns.

One free Walk-ilates class with each MBT purchase!

Contact Ellie Herman (ellie@elliehermanpilates.com) for Walk-ilates workshops and Teacher Training both nationally and internationally.

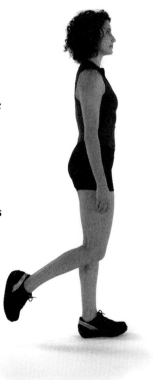

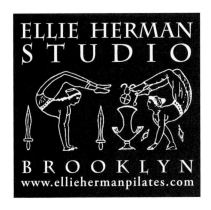

CHANGING THE WORLD ONE VERTEBRATE AT A TIME